The ABC Approach
to Preventing the Sexual
Transmission of HIV

Common and Answers

**Christian Connections
for International Health**

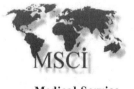

**Medical Service
Corporation International**

The ABC Approach
to Preventing the Sexual Transmission of HIV
Common Questions and Answers

Additional·copies of this document can be obtained from CCIH for distribution to your staff, colleagues, project personnel, church or other leaders who might benefit from this information about the ABC approach. Also, for ideas on addressing the ABC approach in conferences, workshops, or training programs, contact CCIH.

Christian Connections for International Health
1817 Rupert Street
McLean, VA 22101, USA
Phone: 703-556-0123
Email: ccih@ccih.org
Web: http://www.ccih.org

Medical Service Corporation International
1716 Wilson Boulevard
Arlington, VA 22209, USA
Phone: 703-276-3000
Email: msci@mscionline.com
Web: http://www.mscionline.com

Library of Congress Number: 2006932109
International Standard Book Number: 1-932864-96-2

This document may be cited as follows:

Green EC, Herling A. *The ABC Approach to Preventing the Sexual Transmission of HIV: Common Questions and Answers*. McLean, VA: Christian Connections for International Health and Medical Service Corporation International, 2007.

Table of Contents

Acknowledgements

This document is an initiative of the HIV Prevention and Health Behavior Working Group of Christian Connections for International Health (CCIH), and was produced through a collaborative effort between CCIH and Medical Service Corporation International (MSCI). CCIH is an association of 70 Christian organizations, 10 secular affiliate organizations, and 350 individuals working in international health. CCIH's mission is to promote international health and wholeness from a Christian perspective through providing field-oriented information resources and a forum for discussion, networking, and fellowship to the spectrum of Christian organizations and individuals working in international health. MSCI is a diversified international health and development company. MSCI is involved in the design, implementation and management of technical assistance programs in disease control, environmental health, health services delivery, health education, and psychosocial services.

Edward C. Green, PhD, is the principal author of this publication. Dr. Green is a Senior Research Scientist at the Harvard School of Public Health and the Director of the AIDS Prevention Research Project at the Harvard Center for Population and Development Studies. He currently serves on both the Presidential Advisory Council for HIV/AIDS and the Advisory Council, Office of AIDS Research, U.S. Department of Health and Human Services. For the past 20 years, Dr. Green has developed, evaluated, and implemented HIV/AIDS prevention programs in Africa, Asia, Latin America, and the Caribbean. He is the author of *Rethinking AIDS Prevention: Learning from Successes in Developing Countries* (Praeger, 2003), *AIDS and STDs in Africa* (1994) and other books.

Allison Herling, MSPH, also contributed significantly to the writing of this document. Ms. Herling is a Research Fellow at the AIDS Prevention Research Project at the Harvard Center for Population and Development Studies. She has worked for CCIH, Catholic Relief Services, the USAID-funded Synergy Project and MSCI. Her work has taken her to Uganda, Kenya, Morocco, Jamaica, Zimbabwe, and Mozambique.

This document was reviewed and refined by the members of CCIH's HIV Prevention and Health Behavior Working Group. The Working Group would like to thank the following individuals for their review of this document. Their expertise contributed greatly to the development of this document, although their inclusion on this list does not imply endorsement of the final contents of this document.

- Dorothy Brewster-Lee, MD, MPH, Vice-President, Christian Connections for International Health
- Cynthia Calla, MD, MPH, Executive Director, LifeRise AIDS Resources
- Ken Casey, Special Representative to the President, HIV/AIDS Hope Initiative, World Vision International
- Sharon Franzén, Program Associate, Christian Connections for International Health
- Helene D. Gayle MD, MPH, President and CEO, CARE USA
- Szymon Grzelak, PhD, Vice-President, Homo Homini Charles de Foucauld Foundation, Poland
- Norman Hearst, MD, MPH, Professor, University of California, San Francisco
- Douglas Kirby, PhD, Senior Research Scientist, ETR Associates
- Hanna Klaus, MD, Executive Director, Natural Family Planning Center of Washington, D.C. and Teen STAR Program
- Purnima Mane, Director, Policy, Evidence and Partnerships, Joint United Nations Programme on HIV/AIDS (UNAIDS)

- Ray Martin, Executive Director, Christian Connections for International Health
- W. Henry Mosley, MD, MPH, Professor, Department of Population, Reproductive and Family Health, Johns Hopkins Bloomberg School of Public Health
- Carrie Miller, HIV/AIDS Technical Advisor, Program Quality and Support Department, Catholic Relief Services
- Elaine M. Murphy, PhD, Scholar-in-Residence, Population Reference Bureau
- Charles Ndungu, Program Officer, Center for Democracy and Development, University of Massachusetts
- Julie Pulerwitz, ScD, Research Director, Horizons Program/ Population Council, seconded from PATH
- Gordon Raley, Director of Public Policy, Family Health International
- Ed Scholl, Deputy Director YouthNet Program, Family Health International
- Will Story, MPH, Child Survival and Health Technical Advisor, Christian Reformed World Relief Committee
- Laura van Vuuren, HIV and AIDS Senior Technical Advisor, Northwest Medical Teams

Conflict of Interest Statement

Dr. Green is a Senior Research Scientist and Ms. Herling is a Research Fellow at Harvard University. Harvard University does not present a conflict of interest *vis-à-vis* the subject matter of this publication, nor does CCIH or MSCI.

Comments and Suggestions

The authors and the CCIH HIV Prevention and Health Behavior Working Group invite your comments, criticisms, and suggestions for future publications and projects. You may contact Dr. Green at egreendc@aol.com, and Ms. Herling at aherling@gmail.com. The CCIH HIV Prevention and Health Behavior Working Group can be contacted at ccih@ccih.org. You may also send comments by mail to Christian Connections for International Health (1817 Rupert St., McLean, VA, 22101, USA), or to Medical Service Corporation International (1716 Wilson Blvd., Arlington, VA, 22209, USA).

Abbreviations and Acronyms

ABC	Abstain, Be faithful, or use Condoms
ABCplus	an HIV prevention approach that emphasizes ABC behaviors *and* addresses the effects of gender, poverty, violence, stigma, and discrimination on sexual behavior
ANC	Antenatal clinic
ART	Antiretroviral therapy
ARV	Antiretroviral drug
CCIH	Christian Connections for International Health
DHS	Demographic and Health Surveys
FBO	Faith-based organization
MC	Male circumcision
MSCI	Medical Service Corporation International
OGAC	Office of the U.S. Global AIDS Coordinator
PEPFAR	President's Emergency Plan for AIDS Relief (Emergency Plan)
PLWA	People living with HIV/AIDS
STI	Sexually transmitted infection
UNAIDS	Joint United Nations Programme on HIV/AIDS
UNFPA	United Nations Population Fund
USAID	U.S. Agency for International Development
VCT	Voluntary counseling and testing
WHO	World Health Organization

Introduction

The ABC approach—Abstain, Be faithful, or use Condoms— has been the subject of much attention and controversy in recent years, as it has become the policy of the largest AIDS relief plan in the history of the pandemic. In January 2003, the United States pledged $15 billion to global AIDS under the President's Emergency Plan for AIDS Relief (PEPFAR). The U.S. Agency for International Development (USAID) had recently adopted the ABC approach as the model of HIV prevention for generalized epidemics, using Uganda's success as a model. In 2003, PEPFAR also adopted the ABC approach. The first PEPFAR prevention strategy document to be released announced that "risk elimination" would be the "cornerstone" of prevention under PEPFAR.[1] Risk elimination, also called risk avoidance, refers to sexual abstinence and to mutual fidelity between two uninfected sex partners. Risk reduction, on the other hand, refers to strategies such as condom usage that reduce but do not eliminate the risk of sexual transmission. PEPFAR, through the ABC approach, would combat AIDS both ways. The Office of the U.S. Global AIDS Coordinator

---

[1] Office of the United States Global Aids Coordinator for AIDS Relief. *The President's Emergency Plan for AIDS Relief: U.S. Five-Year Global HIV/AIDS Strategy.* Washington, DC, Feb 2004.

(OGAC) later released further guidance on the ABC approach.[2] Although this guidance has clarified the prevention approach to be followed by programs under PEPFAR, considerable confusion and controversy remain. The evidence for and appropriate application of the ABC approach to HIV prevention remain widely misinterpreted and misunderstood.

The HIV Prevention and Health Behavior Working Group of Christian Connections for International Health (CCIH) has recognized a need for a document that explains the ABC approach to HIV prevention, clearly presents the evidence for such an approach, and responds to common critiques with empirical evidence. CCIH itself has decided to use the term "ABCplus" to denote an HIV prevention approach that emphasizes ABC behaviors *and* addresses the effects of gender, poverty, violence, stigma, and discrimination on sexual behavior. This term in fact captures the full program that Uganda pioneered. However, we will use the widely-recognized term "ABC" in this document because that is the term being debated, even if "ABC" is sometimes presented as something quite different from the actual approach that Uganda developed beginning in the latter 1980s.

It is not the intention of the Working Group, CCIH, or the authors of this document to be provocative or polemical, although criticisms will be addressed and answered. The position developed in this document reflects major elements of the policies of PEPFAR, USAID, and the "Consensus Statement" published in the medical journal *The Lancet* on December 1, 2004 and endorsed by over 150 public health experts world-

---

[2] Office of the United States Global AIDS Coordinator for AIDS Relief. *ABC Guidance for United States Government In-Country Staff and Implementing Partners Applying the ABC Approach to Preventing Sexually Transmitted HIV Infections within The President's Emergency Plan for AIDS Relief.* Washington, DC, Mar 2005.

wide and the president of Uganda.[3] Stated simply, this position is that all three components of the ABC approach are necessary, and that the application of this approach will vary according to the target groups. UNAIDS and some other donors and AIDS organizations have also publicly endorsed all the elements of ABC, with varying levels of priority given to the respective elements according to the type and stage of an HIV/AIDS epidemic.

The ABC approach addresses the sexual transmission of HIV and has proven most effective in generalized epidemics, as opposed to epidemics concentrated among high-risk groups. Therefore, this document will address only the sexual transmission of HIV and will focus on transmission within generalized epidemics, predominantly those in sub-Saharan Africa (sometimes referred to here simply as Africa). Eastern and Southern Africa are by far the highest HIV prevalence regions in the world and bear the greatest burden of the global HIV/AIDS pandemic. Africa also provides the clearest examples of the success of an ABC approach in turning the tide of generalized epidemics, and of AB behavior changes impacting HIV prevalence at the population level.

We wish to note that 25 years into the AIDS pandemic it is becoming increasingly clear that most epidemics, including the fast-growing epidemics of Eastern Europe and the Central Asian republics, are not generalized. Even in Africa, not all countries and regions follow the pattern of a generalized epidemic. Most of the West African epidemics—such as those of Senegal, the Gambia, Mali, Niger, Guinea and even Ghana—are not really turning out to be generalized. Population-based sero-surveys are showing that prevalence in all of these countries ranges from under 1% to just over 2%, and most HIV infections occur among

---

[3] Halperin DT, Steiner MJ, Cassell MM et al. The Time Has Come for Common Ground on Preventing Sexual Transmission of HIV. *The Lancet* 2004; 364: 1913–1915.

vulnerable groups such as sex workers and their clients. These transmission dynamics resemble the epidemics of most parts of the world, where transmission also occurs mainly within vulnerable groups.

World Bank AIDS expert David Wilson has urged that we move forward from a conventional threshold-based definition (in which an epidemic is considered generalized if prevalence is over 1%, an arbitrary cut-off) as this obscures real understanding of HIV transmission patterns. He suggests alternative, *transmission*-based definitions, namely: "Epidemics are concentrated if transmission occurs mostly among vulnerable groups and if protecting vulnerable groups would protect wider society. Conversely, epidemics are generalized if transmission occurs mainly outside vulnerable groups and would continue despite effective vulnerable group interventions."[4]

The use of these definitions along with recognition that most HIV epidemics are concentrated reminds us that interventions for what have been called the universally vulnerable groups—sex workers (usually female), injecting drug users, and men who have sex with men—remain an essential part of AIDS prevention. Interventions for these vulnerable groups can include risk reduction measures such as condom supply and promotion as well as interventions that help to eliminate high-risk behaviors. Encouraging men who have sex with men to practice faithfulness, helping girls and women leave sex work, preventing drug addiction in the general population, and helping addicts break out of addiction are all needed interventions that have been tried in various settings. Promoting fidelity and abstinence to the general population should also always be part of an overall prevention strategy, whatever the type of epidemic.

---

[4] Wilson D. *A Monitoring and Evaluation Framework for Concentrated Epidemics and Vulnerable Populations.* Washington, DC: The World Bank, 2005.

The summary section of this document contains a list of questions and short answers. This section is followed by a list of the same questions, with more in-depth answers. The short answers are intended for the reader who wants a quick overview of issues surrounding the ABC approach. For those who want a more in-depth understanding, the full answers provide a more thorough explanation, including relevant research and data.

We hope that all readers will gain a greater understanding of the ABC approach through this document, and that the power of this approach to sharply reduce the sexual transmission of HIV/AIDS within generalized epidemics will be clearly understood.

Note on the ABC Abbreviation

Uganda did not actually call its program ABC prior to the late 1990s. Its distinctive approach to AIDS prevention had no particular name. At this time the World Health Organization (WHO) and some other international organizations involved in AIDS sometimes used ABC to outline what people *ought* to do, but in practice few actual resources went to the A or B components. Uganda and Senegal were among the only exceptions to this unwritten rule or tacit agreement among major donors. By the late 1990s, attempts to describe Uganda's unusual program, such as by the first author of the present book, used ABC as a convenient abbreviation (note it is not an acronym) since Uganda did in fact emphasize A and B before advising C. The condom option was for those who would not or could not practice abstinence or faithful monogamy or faithful polygamy ("zero grazing").

Yet Uganda's response to AIDS involved more than addressing ABC behaviors. Uganda in fact pioneered approaches towards reducing stigma, bringing discussion of sexual behavior out into the open, involving HIV-infected people in public education, persuading individuals and couples to be tested and counseled, improving the status of women, involving religious organizations, enlisting the help of traditional healers, and much more. To recognize the role of these factors, some groups have decided to use the term ABCplus. CCIH has introduced the term to remind the world of other interventions that help facilitate ABC behavioral changes (or more often, if we go by the data, behavior *maintenance.*) In 2005, the Uganda AIDS Commission decided to re-launch Uganda's ABC approach as "ABC plus" in order to "comprehensively accommodate the existing and emerging challenges" in HIV prevention[5] and include consideration of "all environments and factors that influence ABC behaviours as well as other HIV prevention intervention strategies, such as prevention of mother-to-child transmission (PMTCT)."[6]

ABC is a convenient shorthand for discussing specific behaviors and interventions targeting these behaviors. Also in its favor, ABC is immediately understood not only by those who work in HIV/AIDS and related professional fields, but also by the rank and file in Africa and other resource poor areas of the world. ABC recognizes the contributing role of all three interventions and behaviors, including condom use. It

---

[5]   Uganda AIDS Commission. *Is the ABC Message Still Effective in Contemporary Uganda: Summary Synthesis Report of the Uganda Think Tank on AIDS, 3rd Session, 14th July 2005.* Kampala, Uganda: Uganda AIDS Commission, 2005. Available at http://www.aidsuganda.org/ UTTA%20documentation/UTTA%203/UTTA%203%20report.pdf (accessed 8 Jan 2007).

[6]   John Rwomushana, Uganda AIDS Commission, personal communication, 12 Jan 2007.

implicitly separates discourse from "abstinence only" posi-
tions, in spite of persistent attempts to confuse the issue and
misrepresent AB interventions as "abstinence only" and to
call ABC an American or Bush Administration model or
approach. This linkage of the three interventions in ABC helps
those committed to condoms accept the A and B options, and
those committed to AB interventions accept condoms. ABC
implies equivalence among the elements, although their rank
order reflects the priority in which they arguably ought to be
considered, since it is a basic public health maxim that avoiding a risk is inherently better than reducing a risk. ABC also
implies a balanced approach, a menu of options instead of
only one or two. It signals that promotion of abstinence and
mutual fidelity (a newer approach, at least for major donors)
is being added to risk reduction (an older, more established
approach in AIDS prevention), and that *both* approaches are
needed, depending on the age, circumstances, and risk category of those targeted.

ABC further implies getting down to basics, to fundamen-
tals, to simplicity, and to primary prevention, which has been
curiously missing from HIV/AIDS prevention (an anomaly
among diseases), if we are speaking of allocation of funds from
major donors. ABC further implies that AIDS prevention need
not be rocket science as long as it is willing to deal with the
behaviors epidemiologically known to impact HIV transmission. The sexual transmission of HIV can be prevented by
blocking the reproduction rate of infection in three ways: (a) by
avoiding the exposure to risk (through sexual abstinence, or
mutual faithfulness among uninfected partners), (b) by *reducing* the frequency of exposure to risk (through reduction in
numbers of partners), and (c) by *reducing* the efficiency of HIV

transmission (by condom use and by male circumcision in heterosexually-driven epidemics). As noted above, avoiding exposure to risk is always preferable to risk reduction. While reducing one's number of sexual partners can reduce risk, the goal of B interventions should be mutual fidelity (within monogamous or polygamous unions), which when practiced between HIV-negative partners completely eliminates the risk of sexual transmission of HIV.

Summary of Common Questions and Answers about the ABC Approach to HIV Prevention

1. What is the ABC approach to HIV prevention? (p. 21)

"A" stands for Abstaining from sex, "B" stands for Being faithful (fidelity), and "C" stands for Condom use. The ABC approach employs population-specific interventions that emphasize abstinence for youth and other unmarried persons, including delay of sexual debut; mutual faithfulness (sometimes measured as reduction in number of sexual partners) for sexually active adults; and correct and consistent use of condoms by those whose behavior places them at risk for transmitting or becoming infected with HIV. The ABCplus approach is an HIV prevention approach that emphasizes ABC behaviors *and* addresses the effects of gender, poverty, violence, stigma, and discrimination on sexual behavior. As will be seen, in all cases in which an ABC approach has been successful in reducing HIV prevalence within a population, "plus" elements such as increased gender equality and decreased stigma and discrimination have also been present.

2. What evidence is there for an ABC approach? (p. 22)

An ABC approach has been shown to be effective in generalized epidemics—that is, epidemics in which most infections are found in the general population, rather than limited to high-risk groups such as intravenous (IV) drug users or sex workers. Uganda provides the clearest case study of a successful ABC approach. HIV prevalence peaked in Uganda at 15% in 1991, and decreased to 5% by 2001.[1] During this period, abstinence and age of sexual debut increased among youth and condom use increased.[2] Most critically, B behaviors (fidelity and reduction in number of sexual partners) increased, and the decrease in multiple sexual partnerships and networks appears to have been the most important determinant of the reduction in HIV incidence.[3] Other countries in which elements of an ABC approach seem to have contributed to a reduction in HIV prevalence include Senegal, Jamaica, Thailand, Zambia, the Dominican Republic, and, most recently, Kenya, Zimbabwe, and Rwanda.

3. Aren't all parts of the ABC approach important? Why do proponents of the ABC approach often emphasize abstinence and fidelity and not consider condom use an equally valid choice? (p. 27)

According to a 2004 statement published in *The Lancet* and endorsed by 150 public health experts, all the elements of the ABC approach are necessary, "although the emphasis placed on individual elements needs to vary according to the target population."[4] For youth, the first priority should be to encourage abstinence or delay of sexual debut. For adults, the first priority should be to promote mutual fidelity with an uninfected partner. Finally, for people at high risk of exposure to HIV, the first priority should be to promote consistent condom use.

4. Are condoms effective against HIV/AIDS? (p. 29)

Condoms are estimated to be between 80% and 90% effective against HIV when used consistently and correctly—that is, to

---

[1]   Green EC, Nantulya V, Stoneburner R, Stover J. *What Happened in Uganda? Declining HIV Prevalence, Behavior Change, and the National Response.* Washington, DC: USAID, 2002. Available at http://www.usaid.gov/our_work/global_health/aids/Countries/africa/uganda_report.pdf (accessed 8 Apr 2006).

[2]   Demographic and Health Surveys (DHS). Available at www.measuredhs.com.

[3]   Green et al., 2002.

[4]   Halperin, Steiner et al., 2004.

reduce HIV transmission by 80% to 90% compared to non-use.[5,6] Promotion of condoms alone has not been shown to be an effective strategy to lower infection rates in generalized epidemics, such as those found in Africa.[7] Condoms have been shown to reduce HIV prevalence in concentrated epidemics, as in Thailand and Cambodia, where most HIV infections are found among high-risk groups. High levels of consistent condom use have been achieved among certain high-risk groups. For populations other than high-risk groups, inconsistent condom use is the norm rather than the exception. As a 2003 study concluded, "There is little evidence that sometimes (but not always) using condoms provides any protection as compared to not using condoms at all."[8]

5. Should condoms be promoted only to high-risk populations such as sex workers and truck drivers? Doesn't everyone need condoms? (p. 36)

Condoms can be promoted to anyone and everyone, yet many years of experience provides persuasive evidence that those outside of high-risk groups are unlikely to use them consistently. Furthermore, mounting evidence suggests that inconsistent condom use does not protect people, possibly because risk compensation or disinhibition may cause condom users to take greater risks in their sexual behavior. Guidance from the Office of the U.S. Global AIDS Coordinator (OGAC) suggests that condom promotion be targeted to high-risk groups, following Uganda's successful approach during the 1990s. Those engaging in high-risk behaviors (such as commercial sex, sex with multiple partners, or sex with a person known or likely to be infected with HIV) are more likely to

---

[5]   Weller S, Davis K. Condom effectiveness in reducing heterosexual HIV transmission. *Cochrane Database Systematic Review* 2002; (1): CD003255.

[6]   Hearst N, Chen S. Condom Promotion for AIDS Prevention in the Developing World: Is it Working? *Studies in Family Planning* 2004; 35(1): 39–47.

[7]   Hearst & Chen, 2004.

[8]   Hearst N, Chen S. Condoms for AIDS Prevention in the Developing World: A Review of the Scientific Literature. Geneva: UNAIDS, 12 Jan 2003, p. 31.

use condoms, especially when condoms are promoted effectively and made readily available. Promoting condom use to those with high-risk behaviors is also strategic in that they are more likely to be "core transmitters" within a population.

> Risk compensation and disinhibition refer to the tendency for a perception of reduced risk to make risk taking more attractive. People adjust their behavior in response to the increased sense of personal safety that comes with protective behaviors such as wearing a seatbelt or using a condom.

6. Does providing information about condoms lead to earlier or increased sexual activity among youth? (p. 40)

Studies from developed countries as well as developing countries have found that providing information about condoms in sex and HIV education programs that primarily emphasize abstinence does not lead to earlier or more frequent sexual activity among youth.[9] Such sex education programs can, in fact, delay sex and increase abstinence (as well as lead to greater condom use among sexually active youth). Demographic and Health Surveys (DHS) data show that the majority of adults in sub-Saharan Africa think that youth should be taught about the use of condoms to prevent HIV/AIDS.[10]

7. Does the ABC approach demand an unrealistic standard of behavior? (p. 43)

Many factors can limit or take away a person's ability to practice abstinence, faithfulness, or consistent condom use. These factors include poverty, illiteracy, instability and displace-

---

[9]   Kirby D, Laris BA, Rolleri L. *Impact of Sex and HIV Curriculum-Based Education Programs in Schools and Communities on Sexual Behaviors of Youth. Youth Research Working Paper No. 2*. Arlington, VA: FHI/YouthNet, 2005.
[10]   DHS. Available at www.measuredhs.com.

ment, and gender inequity. Yet data show that more than half of African youth aged 15 to 19 abstained from premarital sex last year, and the great majority of sexually active adults were faithful, meaning that they did not report more than one sex partner in the last year.[11] Not only are most Africans practicing A and B behaviors, but 93% of Africans aged 15 to 49 are *not* HIV infected. According to UNAIDS, sub-Saharan Africa now has an average adult HIV prevalence rate of 5.9%, down from 6.0% in 2004.[12] Furthermore, some of the strongest evidence for effectiveness of an ABC approach comes from situations in which there were high levels of poverty, illiteracy, and instability, such as Uganda during the late 1980s and early 1990s.

8. Is the ABC approach unrealistic for women? (p. 48)

It is a tragic fact that some women who have practiced pre-marital abstinence and marital fidelity have nevertheless become infected by unfaithful spouses or partners. According to the United Nations Population Fund (UNFPA), 60–80% of HIV-positive women in Africa have been infected by their husbands.[13,14] In addition, women may be victims of rape and sexual violence, including violence within marriage, and may be made vulnerable by poverty or other circumstances. The ABC approach should go hand in hand with addressing gender inequity. Furthermore,

---

[11] DHS. Available at www.measuredhs.com.

[12] UNAIDS. *UNAIDS/WHO AIDS Epidemic Update 2006*. Geneva: UNAIDS, 2006. Available at http://www.unaids.org/en/HIV_data/epi2006 (accessed 23 Jan 2007).

[13] UNFPA. *State of World Population 2005: The Promise of Equality: Gender Equity, Reproductive Health, and the Millennium Development Goals*. New York: UNFPA, 2005. Available at http://www.unfpa.org/swp/2005/pdf/ (accessed 18 May 2006).

[14] Norman Hearst of University of California, San Francisco is skeptical of this figure: "It doesn't fit the reality that, in most generalized epidemics, many women get infected in their teens, with much higher rates of infection among young women than young men. Perhaps 80% are in a monogamous relationship at the time they *discover* they are infected. The 80% figure also doesn't jive with the fact that, in most settings, discordant couples tend to be about 50% male positive, 50% female positive." Personal communication, 22 May 2006.

there must be consciousness raising among women and girls so that they realize and exercise the control that they do have over their sexual lives. Although some women may be unable to practice abstinence, ensure mutual fidelity, or use condoms (given their relative lack of power in patriarchal societies), available data show that the majority of women in Africa exercise more freedom of individual choice than is often attributed to them. Last year, two-thirds of unmarried girls and women in Africa (ages 15 to 24) practiced abstinence.[15] The majority of women in Africa—ranging from 71% of women in Zimbabwe to 87% of women in Rwanda—report that a woman is justified in refusing sex with her husband for reasons such as knowing that he has a sexually transmitted infection (STI).[16,17] The belief in the West that most African women have few or no choices or options in matters of sexual behavior is not supported empirically.

9. Does the ABC approach consider local realities such as gender and social inequalities, poverty, and cultural impediments to behavior change? (p. 51)

An ABC approach focuses on what an individual can do to change (or maintain) behavior, and thereby avoid or reduce risk of infection, while also recognizing that not all individuals have control over their sexual behavior. An ABC approach incorporates broader goals such as advancing women, increasing access to education, and decreasing poverty. Individual behavioral

---

[15] DHS. Available at www.measuredhs.com.

[16] DHS data, cited in Murphy E, Greene ME, Duong T. *Defending the ABCs: A Feminist Perspective on AIDS Prevention*. Presentation at African Successes: Can Behavior-Based Solutions Make a Crucial Contribution to HIV Prevention in Sub-Saharan Africa? Munyonyo, Uganda, 17-20 Dec 2006.

[17] Even in countries in which a great majority of women report that a woman is justified in refusing sex with her husband, other data point to women's continued vulnerability. According to DHS data, a significant minority of women in Africa agree that a husband is justified in hitting or beating his wife for reasons such as burning the food, arguing with him, or refusing to have sex with him. Over half of women in Rwanda and Uganda believe that a husband is justified in hitting or beating his wife if she neglects the children.

approaches to the prevention of sexual transmission of HIV should be complemented by larger community and societal responses. Yet, these important broader societal and structural goals may not be achievable in the short or even medium term. In Uganda and other countries, HIV prevention has been successful even though these broader goals (although pursued) have not been fully met.

10. Is the ABC approach overly simplistic? (p. 53)

Some argue that the ABC approach is overly simplistic and that we need to go "beyond ABC" to an approach that includes other interventions such as voluntary counseling and testing (VCT), treatment of HIV and other STIs, destigmatization, reducing poverty, increasing political openness, and educating women and improving their status. These interventions should be promoted vigorously both because they are critical matters of justice and human rights and because they likely create an environment that encourages changes in sexual behavior. Yet they do not in themselves directly prevent the sexual transmission of HIV. They are effective only to the extent that they lead to increased practice of A, B, or C behaviors. Data show that expanding access to VCT does not necessarily reduce HIV prevalence in a population.[18, 19, 20, 21] In some countries HIV

[18] Matovu JKB, Kigozi G, Nalugoda F. *Repetitive VCT, Sexual Risk Behavior and HIV-Incidence in Rakai, Uganda.* Presentation at the Uganda Virus Research Institute, Entebbe, Uganda, 28 Nov 2003.

[19] Weinhardt LS, Carey MP, Johnson BT, Bickham NL. Effects of HIV Counseling and Testing on Sexual Risk Behavior: A Meta-Analytic Review of Published Research, 1985–1997. *American Journal of Public Health* 1999; 89: 1397–1405.

[20] Wolitski R, MacGowan R, Higgins D, Jorgensen C. The Effects of HIV Counseling and Testing on Risk-Related Practices and Help-Seeking Behavior. *AIDS Education and Prevention* 1997; 9(Suppl B): 52–67.

[21] Glick P. *Scaling up HIV Voluntary Counseling and Testing in Africa: What Can Evaluation Studies Tell Us about Potential Prevention Impacts?* Strategies and Analysis for Growth and Access (SAGA) Working Paper. Cornell University, Mar 2005.

prevalence rises—rather than falls—with income level.[22] We might find political leadership, open discussion of HIV/AIDS, or other factors conducive to fighting AIDS, yet no decline in HIV transmission within a country. The only way to directly influence the sexual transmission of HIV is through changes in sexual behavior. Incorporating a range of other approaches in an HIV prevention strategy can be helpful if these approaches are designed to lead clearly to changes in sexual behavior. If they are advocated instead of a strong focus on ABC-related sexual behavior changes, they are not likely to be successful.

11. Does the ABC approach contribute to stigmatization and marginalization of people living with HIV/AIDS (PLWAs)? (p. 58)

People Living with HIV/AIDS (PLWAs) are often leaders in the fight against HIV/AIDS. In many African countries, networks of PLWAs are leaders in advocating for behavior change, including an ABC approach. Some people may feel marginalized or stigmatized by an ABC approach and may face social disapproval for either engaging in or *not* engaging in A, B, or C behaviors. Yet to object to the promotion of abstinence and faithfulness because some will not or cannot abstain or be faithful denies information and support to the majority of the population that does, in fact, already practice AB behaviors.

12. Has PEPFAR imposed the ABC approach on people in the developing world? (p. 59)

The President's Emergency Plan for AIDS Relief (PEPFAR) has adopted an ABC approach for generalized HIV/AIDS epidemics, following the Ugandan model of a balanced ABC approach that was successful in reducing HIV prevalence. Uganda's response to HIV/AIDS—the ABC approach—was an

---

[22] Shelton JD, Cassell MM, Adetunji J. Is Poverty or Wealth at the Root of HIV? *The Lancet* 2005; 366: 1057–1058.

indigenous response to the threat of HIV/AIDS and was not an American invention. Africans, and particularly Ugandans, should be given the credit for developing an approach that is culturally relevant, low cost, sustainable and successful.

13. Is PEPFAR promoting abstinence and faithfulness at the expense of condoms? (p. 61)

PEPFAR supports a comprehensive ABC approach, and the U.S. Government is the largest single supplier of condoms worldwide. Under PEPFAR, annual condom procurement has been steadily rising, and the Office of the Global AIDS Coordinator estimates that in 2005 the U.S. Government shipped more than 612 million condoms to Africa, Asia, and Latin America, the greatest annual figure since 1995.[23,24] In spite of this, it is often alleged that PEPFAR is promoting an "abstinence-only" strategy. This is inaccurate both because of PEPFAR's continued support of condoms for at-risk populations and because the ABC approach emphasizes fidelity as well as abstinence (and is therefore not abstinence-only).

14. A recent study suggested that condoms and mortality from AIDS—and not abstinence and faithfulness—had caused HIV prevalence to decline in Uganda. Does this mean that an ABC approach didn't work in Uganda after all? (p. 63)

A 2005 paper presented by Wawer, Gray et al.[25] was widely interpreted as proving that condoms and mortality from

[23] Chaya N, Amen K, Fox M. *Condoms Count: Meeting the Need in the Era of HIV/AIDS: 2004 Data Update.* 2004. Population Action International. Available at http://www.populationaction.org/resources/publications/condomscount/downloads/2004updateInsert_final.pdf (accessed 8 Apr 2006).

[24] Donnelly J. U.S. Condom Policy in Africa Targets "High-Risk" Areas. *Boston Globe*, 8 Sept 2005.

[25] Wawer MJ, Gray R et al. *Declines in HIV Prevalence in Uganda: Not as Simple as ABC.* Presentation at Conference on Retroviruses and Opportunistic Infections. Boston, 22 Feb 2005.

AIDS—and not abstinence and faithfulness—were responsible for Uganda's decline in HIV prevalence. A more careful analysis of these same data is that there had been major changes in behavior toward abstinence and faithfulness prior to the study period (1995–2004). This led to a decrease in HIV incidence prior to 1995 and a corresponding decrease in HIV prevalence after 1995. Although HIV prevalence declined between 1995 and 2004, incidence did not, despite the fact that condom use was increasing. This suggested that other protective behaviors were on the decline. In fact, between 1995 and 2004 A and B behaviors declined.

Incidence is the number of new cases of a disease over a certain period. Prevalence is the proportion of a population infected with a disease at a given time.

15. Even if the ABC approach did work in Uganda, is there evidence that it could work in other countries? (p. 65)

An ABC approach has been implemented to varying degrees in Senegal, Jamaica, Zambia, Kenya, and Thailand, all with positive results. Kenya may provide the most recent example of a successful ABC approach. HIV prevalence in Kenya peaked in the late 1990s at 10% and had declined to 7% by 2003.[26] During this period, Kenya also saw significant increases in A and B behaviors and a smaller increase in condom use reported at last higher-risk sex.[27]

---

[26] UNAIDS, 2005a.
[27] DHS. Available at www.measuredhs.com.

16. In mature epidemics,[28] a large percentage of new HIV infection can occur in serodiscordant couples. How can an ABC approach curb transmission among these couples? (p. 70)

Condom usage rates among married or regular partners are typically low, with less than 5% of regular partners reporting consistent use.[29] Couples' counseling may increase usage rates among discordant couples,[30] but A and B messages can also have great relevance. Serodiscordant couples report abstinence as well as condom usage as strategies to avoid infection, and research has shown that many HIV-negative females would prefer abstinence had their partners not refused.[31] Furthermore, to sustain or expand an epidemic, the "reproductive number" (Ro, used by epidemiologists) must be greater than 1, meaning that an infected person must infect more than one other person.[32] Thus, to avoid further transmission of HIV, a B message that strongly discourages extramarital partners is vital.

---

[28] A mature epidemic is one in which infections have moved beyond the rapid infection of the very susceptible.

[29] Norman Hearst, personal communication, 16 June 2005.

[30] Allen S, Meinzen-Derr J, Kautzman M et al. Sexual Behavior of HIV Discordant Couples after HIV Counseling and Testing. *AIDS* 2003; 17(5): 733–740.

[31] Bunnell RE, Nassozi J, Marum E et al., Living with Discordance: Knowledge, Challenges, and Prevention Strategies of HIV-Discordant Couples in Uganda. *AIDS Care* 2005; 17(8): 999–1012.

[32] Cohen MS, Eron JJ. Sexual HIV Transmission and Its Prevention. *Continuing Medical Education Series*; 27 June 2001. Available at http://www.medscape.com.

Common Questions and Answers about the ABC Approach to HIV Prevention

1. What is the ABC approach to HIV prevention?

"A" stands for Abstaining from sex, "B" stands for Being faithful (fidelity), and "C" stands for Condom use. The ABC approach employs population-specific interventions that emphasize abstinence for youth and other unmarried persons, including delay of sexual debut; mutual faithfulness (sometimes measured as reduction in number of sexual partners) for sexually active adults; and correct and consistent use of condoms by those whose behavior places them at risk for transmitting or becoming infected with HIV. The ABC approach offers a menu of options rather than a one-size-fits-all solution. In the words of Ambassador Mark Dybul, U.S. Global AIDS Coordinator:

> To the extent any controversy remains around ABC, I believe it stems from misunderstanding. ABC is not a narrow, one-size-fits-all recipe. It encompasses a wide variety of approaches to the myriad of factors that lead to sexual transmission. The interventions that help people to choose to avoid the risk of HIV infection entirely, or to reduce their risk, vary according to the circumstances of their lives.[1]

The ABCplus approach is an HIV prevention approach that emphasizes ABC behaviors *and* addresses the effects of gender,

---

[1] Testimony before the Subcommittee on National Security, Emerging Threats, and International Relations, Committee on Government Reform, United States House of Representatives. Washington, DC, 6 Sept, 2006.

poverty, violence, stigma, and discrimination on sexual behavior. As will be seen, in all cases in which an ABC approach has been successful in reducing HIV prevalence within a population, "plus" elements such as increased gender equality and decreased stigma and discrimination have also been present.

2. What evidence is there for an ABC approach?

The sexual transmission of HIV can be directly prevented in only three ways: by avoiding the exposure to risk through sexual abstinence; by reducing the risk of exposure through partner faithfulness and reduction in partners; or by blocking the efficiency of transmission through a barrier like a condom. In other words, by practicing A, B, or C. Treatment of sexually transmitted infections (STIs) (including HIV) and male circumcision can also reduce, although not eliminate, the risk of HIV transmission. In the future, vaginal microbicides may also reduce the risk of HIV transmission once a safe and effective drug has been approved for use.

The ABC approach offers risk reduction as well as risk avoidance and options for those at various levels of risk. A broader approach ought to have greater impact than a narrower one, given the variability of human behavior and circumstances. A single preventive approach to something as complex as human sexual behavior will never appeal to all people, let alone influence their behavior. For those who continue to have multiple sexual partners or who are otherwise at risk, the only preventive options may be those classifiable as risk reduction, namely condom use, male circumcision, and appropriate treatment of STIs.

An ABC approach is appropriate for generalized epidemics, which require a different prevention approach than do concentrated epidemics. World Bank AIDS expert David Wilson provides definitions of concentrated and generalized epidemics that point to appropriate interventions. "Epidemics are concentrated if transmission occurs mostly among vulnerable groups and if protecting vulnerable groups would protect wider society. Conversely, epidemics are generalized if transmission occurs mainly outside vulnerable groups and would continue despite effective vulnerable group interventions."[2]

By definition, one cannot impact HIV prevalence in generalized epidemics by promoting risk reduction measures to vulnerable (or high-risk) groups, however successful those interventions might be. What is effective in concentrated epidemics will not necessarily be effective in generalized epidemics. In the United States, Europe, and most of Latin America and Asia, HIV infections are concentrated in a few fairly well defined high-risk groups. In sub-Saharan Africa, most infections are found in the general population. Differences in epidemiological patterns and cultural settings are real and call for different approaches to prevention.

Because Uganda provides the clearest case study of a successful ABC approach, this document makes frequent reference to Uganda. As discussed below, there is also recent evidence for ABC behaviors being associated with reductions in HIV prevalence in Kenya, Zimbabwe, and urban Rwanda.

In Uganda, HIV prevalence decreased from 15% to 5% between 1991 and 2001.[3] During the same period, the following changes in ABC behaviors occurred (Figure 1):

- The proportion of young males age 15–24 reporting premarital sex decreased from 60% in 1989 to 23% in 1995. For females, the decline was from 53% to 16%.[4]

[2] Wilson D. *A Monitoring and Evaluation Framework for Concentrated Epidemics and Vulnerable Populations.* Washington, DC: The World Bank, 2005.
[3] Green et al., 2002.
[4] Bessinger R, Akwara P, Halperin D. *Sexual Behavior, HIV, and Fertility Trends: A Comparative Analysis of Six Countries.* Calverton, MD: ORC Macro, the Measure Project, and United States Agency for International Development. Available at www.cpc.unc.edu/measure/publications/pdf/sr-03-21b.pdf (accessed 3 Jan 2006).

- For all age groups, 41% of males had more than one sex partner in 1989. This declined to 21% by 1995. For females, the decline was from 23% to 9%. The proportion of males reporting three or more sex partners fell from 15% to 3% between 1989 and 1995.[5]

- In 1995, about 6% of sexually active Ugandans used a condom with some regularity. By 2000, this rose to 11% of sexually active Ugandans, or 8% of all Ugandans. In the same period, the percentage of males who used a condom at last higher-risk sex (sex with a non-marital, non-cohabiting partner) increased from 36% to 59%, and the number of females who used a condom at last higher-risk sex increased from 20 to 38%.[6]

Figure 1: ABC Behaviors in Uganda, 1989 to 1995

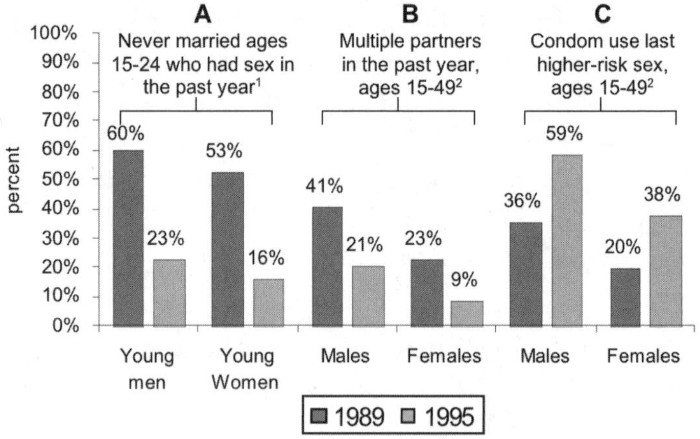

Source: [1]Global Programme on AIDS (GPA), [2]Demographic Health Surveys (DHS)

---

5   DHS. Available at www.measuredhs.com.
6   DHS. Available at www.measuredhs.com.

The main behavior change that occurred in Uganda was a decrease in number of sexual partners and increased monogamy and fidelity (mostly marital fidelity). The decrease in multiple sexual partnerships and networks appears to have been the most important determinant of the reduction in HIV incidence. [7] Although AIDS prevention programs often focus on youth, evidence shows that it is reduction in the number of sexual partners among those who are sexually active—and not abstinence among youth—that is most critical to curbing an AIDS epidemic.[8] Most Ugandans ages 15 to 49 (the age group in which surveys such as DHS measure both behavior and HIV status) were sexually active and faithful, not abstinent. Youth were given information on a range of AIDS prevention options, including condoms, with abstinence (often termed delay of sexual debut) emphasized as the only 100% sure option. Adults were targeted with a "be faithful" message that included slogans such as "love faithfully" and "zero grazing."

Data show that compared to other countries in Africa, it was with regard to B behaviors that Uganda was different.[9] As shown in Figure 2, condom use was not higher in Uganda than in other countries. Rather it is in "be faithful" behaviors that Uganda stands out. There was far less multi-partner sex in Uganda than in other countries, as illustrated in Figure 3.

[7]   Green et al., 2002.

[8]   Shelton JD, Halperin DT, Nantulya V et al. Partner Reduction Is Crucial for Balanced "ABC" Approach to HIV Prevention. *British Medical Journal* 2004; 328: 891–893.

[9]   Stoneburner R, Low-Beer D. Population-Level HIV Declines and Behavioral Risk Avoidance in Uganda. *Science* 2004; 304: 714–718.

Figure 2: Condom Use at Last Sex*

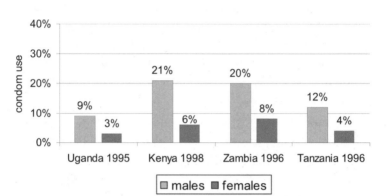

* Percent of sexually active men and women ages 15 to 49 who used a condom at last sex with anyone

Source: Demographic and Health Surveys (DHS)

Figure 3: Multiple Sexual Partnerships*

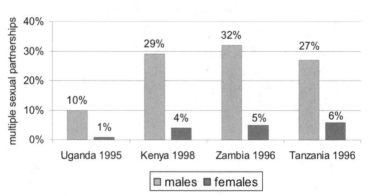

* Percent of sexually active men and women ages 15 to 49 who have had sexual intercourse with more than one partner in the last 12 months

Source: Demographic and Health Surveys (DHS)

There is a clear need for a balance of A, B, and C interventions. Interventions should be targeted for efficiency and likely impact and must take into account crucial differences among target groups. A balanced ABC approach might be implemented in the form of A interventions emphasizing sexual postponement or a return to abstinence for youth; B interventions promoting fidelity or partner reduction to all who are sexually active and especially those not in monogamous relationships (or in polygamous marriages, as was done in Uganda); and C interventions promoting condom use to those at high risk of exposure to HIV infection. People at high risk include those engaging in commercial sex or multiple partnerships, discordant couples and others having sex with a person known or likely to be infected with HIV or another STI, and young people who are sexually active. Yet, these high-risk groups always comprise a minority of any national population. This is true in Africa today, where recent DHS show that the majority of men and women do not report more than one regular sex partner in the previous year.

3. Aren't all parts of the ABC approach important? Why do proponents of the ABC often emphasize abstinence and faithfulness, and not consider condom use an equally valid choice?

According to a statement published in *The Lancet* and endorsed by over 150 public health experts, all the elements of the ABC approach are necessary, "although the emphasis placed on individual elements needs to vary according to the target population."[10] This article states that for youth, the first priority should be to encourage abstinence or delay of sexual debut. For adults, the first priority should be to promote mutual fidelity

---

[10] Halperin, Steiner et al., 2004.

with an uninfected partner. This is especially important, as evidence from countries where HIV has declined suggests that partner reduction and fidelity were the most important behaviors leading to the decline, both in generalized and concentrated epidemics.[11,12] Finally, for people at high risk of exposure to HIV, the first priority should be to promote correct and consistent condom use, along with other approaches such as avoiding high-risk behaviors or partners. Correct information about condoms should be given to all youth and adults, and adults should be encouraged to use condoms correctly and consistently if they have a sexual partner of unknown serostatus. Yet the promotion of condoms to youth and adults who are not in a high-risk category should not precede or supersede efforts to promote abstinence and fidelity.

In appropriately targeting AIDS prevention messages, there is a need to distinguish between individual and public health strategies. This distinction has been made by Dr. Norman Hearst in his evaluation of condom promotion in the developing world. To paraphrase Dr. Hearst: "If I am foolish enough to engage in risky sex, it certainly makes sense for me as an individual to use a condom, since this will greatly reduce my risk of infection. But as a public health strategy, promotion of condoms has had a poor record of producing lower HIV infection rates, especially in generalized epidemics."[13] Similarly, the Phase One report of the USAID ABC Study concluded that A and B behavior changes are necessary for levels of national HIV prevalence to decline in Africa.[14] When abstinence and fidelity are promoted as public health strategies and adopted by large numbers of people, especially in generalized epidemics, HIV prevalence begins to fall.

---

[11] Shelton et al., 2004.

[12] Stoneburner & Low-Beer, 2004.

[13] Hearst N, Chen S. Condom Promotion for AIDS Prevention in the Developing World: Is it Working? *Studies in Family Planning* 2004; 35(1): 39–47.

[14] Bessinger et al., 2003.

4. Are condoms effective against HIV/AIDS?

There are two questions to consider when it comes to condoms and HIV/AIDS. First, how effective are condoms in preventing the transmission of HIV? Second, how successful have condoms been in curbing the spread of HIV within populations?

Condoms are estimated to be between 80% and 90% effective when used consistently and correctly—that is, they reduce HIV transmission by 80% to 90% compared to non-use.[15,16] Condoms can also reduce the risk of many other sexually transmitted infections, the presence of which can increase the transmission efficiency of HIV.

Promotion of condoms alone has not been shown to be an effective strategy to lower infection rates in generalized epidemics, such as those found in Africa. As a 2003 study concluded, "There is little evidence that sometimes (but not always) using condoms provides any protection as compared to not using condoms at all."[17] In a 2004 study, the same researchers concluded, "Especially in the setting of generalized heterosexual transmission, it is unknown what level of condom use in the population is necessary to have a substantial impact on HIV transmission. Indeed, there are no definite examples yet of generalized epidemics that have been turned back by prevention programs based primarily on condom promotion."[18] An article in *The Lancet* similarly stated, "Massive increases in condom use worldwide have not translated into demonstrably improved HIV control in the great majority of countries where they have occurred."[19]

---

[15] Weller & Davis, 2002.

[16] Hearst & Chen, 2004.

[17] Hearst N, Chen S. Condoms for AIDS Prevention in the Developing World: A Review of the Scientific Literature. Geneva: UNAIDS, 12 Jan 2003, p. 31.

[18] Hearst & Chen, 2004.

[19] Richens J, Imrie J, Copas A. Condoms and Seat Belts: The Parallels and the Lessons. *The Lancet* 2000; 29: 400.

Evidence for the effectiveness of condoms in reducing HIV rates at the population level comes from countries like Thailand and Cambodia that have different types of epidemic patterns than are found in Africa. In Thailand, which is considered the world's great condom success story, the epidemic was largely fueled by contact with sex workers. During the early 1990s, the number of men reporting consistent condom use when visiting a sex worker increased from 36% to 71%. During this time period, the number of men reporting premarital or extramarital sex was cut in half and the percentage visiting sex workers was likewise cut in half. [20] All of these trends, along with political support and increased STI control, likely contributed to Thailand's declining HIV incidence during the early 1990s. There is always a lag between incidence and prevalence decline, and data from antenatal clinics (ANCs) showed a decline in HIV prevalence from 2% in 1995 to 1.6% in 2001. [21]

When HIV infections are concentrated among sex workers and their clients, condom promotion is an effective primary strategy, at least for these groups. In Africa, the vast majority of HIV infections occur outside high-risk groups, in the very groups in which condom usage remains stubbornly low. David Wilson of the World Bank recently observed that generalized epidemics will continue "despite effective vulnerable group interventions." [22] In other words, even if sex workers, truck drivers, soldiers, and others at high risk used condoms, epidemics could continue because most infection occurs outside these groups. A different strategy is needed for the majority in the general population—an ABC approach.

Few people are found to use condoms consistently outside high-risk groups. Condom use may be felt to signal a lack of trust

---

[20] Phoolcharoen W. HIV/AIDS Prevention in Thailand: Success and Challenges. *Science* 19 June 1998; 280 (5371): 1873–1874.

[21] Phoolcharoen, 1998.

[22] Wilson, 2005.

within a relationship, to diminish the pleasure of sex, or to be undesirable in other ways. Use of drugs and alcohol can affect a person's ability to use a condom or to use it successfully. Women often lack the power to insist on condom use. Other barriers to condom use include availability and cost. Even in Thailand, condom use among non-sex workers remained relatively low, according to a survey conducted by Family Health International, in which condom use was defined as use during last sexual intercourse. In Bangkok, where condom use among sex workers reached nearly 90% by 1996, reported condom use by women in the general population was only 18.9% in the same year. Only 28.5% of Bangkok sex workers reported using condoms with non-paying sex partners, such as boyfriends. [23]

No country in Africa has ever had rates of consistent condom usage above 5% among married people or regular sexual partners, [24, 25] and usage rates at last intercourse with any type of partner remain relatively low (Table 1). In some countries, condom usage rates among high-risk groups have increased significantly, even as usage rates among the general population have not. In Kenya, between 1998 and 2003, condom use at last higher-risk sex increased from 44% to 47% for men, and from 16% to 24% for women. In the same period, condom use at last sex among all men and women decreased somewhat. [26] This reflected the fact that although condom use was increasing in higher-risk sex, higher-risk sex was on the decline. In other words, an ABC approach was resulting in greater C and especially greater B behaviors.

---

[23] Family Health International. *AIDS Control and Prevention Project: Final Report for the AIDSCAP Program in Thailand November 1991 to September 1996.* Available at http://www.fhi.org/en/HIVAIDS/pub/Archive/aidscapreports/finalreportAIDSCAPthailand/index.htm (accessed 3 Jan 2006).
[24] DHS. Available at www.measuredhs.com.
[25] Hearst N, personal communication, 16 June 2005.
[26] DHS. Available at www.measuredhs.com.

Table 1: Condom Use at Last Sex in Sub-Saharan Africa

Country and year	Percent of sexually active adults ages 15–49 using a condom at last intercourse with any type of partner	
	MALE	FEMALE
Benin 2001	16	4
Burkina Faso 2003	31	9
Cameroon 2004	32	15
Cote d'Ivoire 1998	23	7
Ethiopia 2000	5	1
Ghana 2003	18	9
Guinea 1999	14	3
Kenya 2003	17	5
Malawi 2000	14	5
Mali 2001	10	2
Mozambique 2003	14	6
Namibia 2000	45	28
Nigeria 2003	16	5
Rwanda 2000	6	1
Tanzania 1999[27]	16	8
Togo 1998	19	6
Uganda 2000/01	15	7
Zambia 2001/02	19	12
Zimbabwe 1999	28	9
Average (unweighted)	*19*	*7*

Source: all data from DHS unless otherwise noted

Although correct and consistent condom use may significantly reduce risk of HIV transmission, such usage does not seem to have reached high enough rates in any African country to impact HIV prevalence at a population level. In fact, the number of condoms per male per year in Africa remains low, and in the countries with the highest usage we also see the highest HIV prevalence. In 2000, Shelton and Johnston determined the annual average number of condoms available in several African countries per male aged 15 to 49 years, computing the average

[27] Tanzania Reproductive and Child Health Survey, 1999. Available at www.measuredhs.com.

over a 10-year period.[28] Figure 4 depicts condom availability by country, as well as national HIV prevalence. This figure demonstrates that condom availability in Africa is still very low, largely because of low demand.[29] Yet there are differences among countries. Zimbabwe, Botswana, and South Africa have the highest rates of condom availability but are also among the countries with the highest rates of HIV infection. In contrast, during the unprecedented decline of HIV in Uganda from 1989 through 2000, only four condoms were used per male annually.[30] And as seen in Table 1, the two countries with the lowest condom user rates, Ethiopia and Rwanda, also have low HIV prevalence relative to other countries in East Africa: 4% and 3% respectively.

Figure 4: Average Annual Number of Condoms per Male in Sub-Saharan Africa

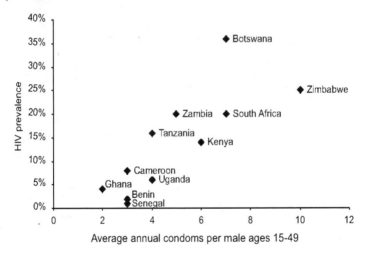

Average annual condoms per male ages 15-49

Source: Shelton and Johnston, 2001

---

[28] Shelton J, Johnston B. Condom Gap in Africa: Evidence from Donor Agencies and Key Informants. *British Medical Journal* 2001; 323: 139.

[29] Longfield K, Agha S, Kusanthan T, et al. *Non-Use of Condoms: What Role Do Supply, Demand, and Acceptance Play in the 'Condom Gap?* Presentation at the International Conference on AIDS and STDs in Africa, Ouagadougou, Burkina Faso, Dec 2001.

[30] Green EC. *Rethinking AIDS Prevention.* Westport, CT: Praeger, 2003.

There are several possible explanations for the relationship between condom use and more HIV infections. The fact that HIV prevalence is highest in the countries with highest condom usage does not necessarily mean that there is a causal relationship or that condom use is in any way contributing to greater HIV prevalence. The range of possible explanations and causal associations include:

1) People who know or suspect they are HIV positive are more likely to use condoms (effect-cause);

2) People who would have more partners anyway are both more likely to use condoms and more likely to be infected (effect-effect);

3) Condom promotion might encourage higher risk sex (cause-effect);

4) Failure to separate out commercial sex (in its various forms) from the data;

5) Failure to fully adjust for other possible confounders.[31]

However, a recent prospective study of Ugandan men published in the *Journal of Acquired Immune Deficiency Syndromes* suggests that condom promotion might in fact encourage higher risk sex ("cause-effect"). In this study, intensive condom promotion was found to lead to increased condom use but also to increased numbers of sex partners, thereby increasing risk of infection. The authors conclude:

> The increase in condom uptake that the intervention produced seems not to have been sufficient to counteract the increase in numbers of sex partners. Although this was not the result we intended or expected, it is consistent with the history of AIDS

---

[31] Hulley SB, Cummings SR, Browner WS et al. *Designing Clinical Research: An Epidemiologic Approach, 2nd Edition.* Philadelphia: Lippincott, Williams & Wilkins, 2001.

prevention efforts in Uganda. Uganda's success in AIDS control seems to have resulted from reductions in numbers of partners, with condoms playing a relatively minor role.[32]

Moreover, the most recent USAID-supported national sample survey of sexual behavior in Uganda, which includes a sero-survey of HIV infection, found that condom users are more likely than non-users to be HIV-infected.[33] This survey compared "condom use ever" (12.2% HIV prevalence) to "never used condom" (6.9% HIV prevalence), and "condom use at last sex in past 12 months" (14.7% HIV prevalence) to "no condom use at last sex in past 12 months" (6.8% HIV prevalence). Only in one condom measure was there no significant difference in HIV prevalence between condom users and non-users. Those who reported condom use and those who reported non-use at last higher-risk sex in past 12 months had the same HIV prevalence (both around 15%), but among those who reported no such higher-risk sex, HIV prevalence was 6.1%.

Similar associations between condom use and higher levels of HIV infection were found by DHS plus sero-surveys in Kenya, Ghana and Tanzania.[34] Studies will have to be done to sort out causal connections. As David Stanton of USAID notes of the new DHS plus sero-surveys:

> The HIV testing technology used in these surveys is unable to establish time of infection. In other words, the result of the test reflects something that could have take place somewhere in an eight to ten year period. Comparing that result to the one-time answer to a survey question needs to be done very carefully. Someone who used condoms consistently and correctly

---

[32] Kajubi P, Kamya MR, Kamya S et al. Increasing Condom Use without Reducing HIV Risk: Results of a Controlled Community Trial in Uganda. *Journal of Acquired Immune Deficiency Syndromes* 2005; 40(1): 77–82.

[33] Ministry of Health (MOH) [Uganda] and ORC Macro. *Uganda HIV/AIDS Sero-behavioural Survey 2004-2005.* Calverton, Maryland, USA: Ministry of Health and ORC Macro, 2006.

[34] DHS. Available at www.measuredhs.com.

in the last 12 months but was infected five years ago doesn't tell us much. I would be very cautious in drawing conclusions from the cross tabulation of HIV test result and survey responses. Even when the data are linked by respondent they are not linked in time let alone cause and effect.[35]

We agree. Yet any positive association between condom use and HIV infection seems to warrant caution in the way condoms are marketed, especially to general populations. A report from Kenya notes:

> [Condom] social marketing plays an important role in increasing demand for and use of all condoms in Kenya, whether they are supplied from the public sector, social marketing, or commercial sources. Mass media campaigns have greatly reduced the societal stigma associated with condoms, which in turn have facilitated their increased availability and use. A generic 'condom efficacy' behaviour change campaign has increased Kenyans' faith in the effectiveness of condoms in preventing disease from 50% to over 80%...[36]

As we market condoms, we need to be careful that we do not unintentionally make risky behaviors seem more attractive.

5. Should condoms be promoted only to high-risk populations such as sex workers and truck drivers? Doesn't everyone need condoms?

Condoms can be promoted to anyone and everyone, yet many years of experience provides persuasive evidence that only those in high-risk groups are likely to use them consistently, especially in rural areas where a steady supply of condoms is problematic. As discussed above, *consistent* condom use in

---

[35] David Stanton, USAID, personal communication, 17 Nov 2006.
[36] National AIDS and STI Control Programme (NASCOP), Ministry of Health, Kenya. *AIDS in Kenya: Trends, Interventions and Impact, 7th ed.* Nairobi: NASCOP, 2005, p. 50.

Africa is rare, and most condom use outside of a very few high-risk groups is *inconsistent*. Mounting evidence suggests that inconsistent condom use does not protect people. In fact, now that DHS include a population-based sero-survey component, it is possible to compare the HIV status of condom users and non-users. In the first countries for which DHS data are available (Tanzania, Kenya, and Ghana), it has been found that condom users were more likely to be infected than non-users, whether the measure is condom use at last sex, last high-risk sex, or last sex with sex workers.[37] These data are being called anomalous, yet they could be explained by factoring in inconsistent and/or incorrect use and the possibility of engaging in higher-risk sex due to disinhibition.[38,39]

Other studies have also provided evidence that inconsistent condom use provides little or no reduced risk of HIV. A study in Rakai, Uganda found that although consistent condom use reduced risk of HIV infection by 63%, irregular condom use did not reduce risk of HIV at all, after adjusting for demographic and behavioral variables.[40] Another recent study found that condom promotion can lead to greater sexual risk taking, which, when combined with inconsistent condom use, results in higher overall risk to HIV. A group of men in Kampala, Uganda participated in a condom promotion program that taught condom technical use skills, encouraged condom use, and provided free condoms. Compared to a control group that received only a brief informational presentation about AIDS, the men in the intervention group did use more condoms. The men in the intervention group also increased their number of sexual partners by 31%, in comparison

---

[37] Annie Cross, Macro International, personal communication, 17 Nov 2005. Also DHS from 2003 onward, available at www.measuredhs.com.

[38] Richens et al., 2000.

[39] Mosley H. Declining HIV in Uganda Cannot Be Explained by Mortality or Condoms (Letter). *British Medical Journal* 2005; 330: 496.

[40] Ahmed S, Lutalo T, Wawer M et al. HIV Incidence and Sexually Transmitted Disease Prevalence Associated with Condom Use: A Population Study in Rakai, Uganda. *AIDS* 2001; 15: 2171–2179.

to the control group, who decreased their number of partners by 17%. The net result was an increase in sexual risk in the intervention group, as "gains in condom use seem to have been offset by increases in the number of sex partners."[41]

We cannot discount the possibility that risk compensation or disinhibition[42] may be causing condom users to take greater risks in their sexual behavior. Ahmed and colleagues found evidence of this in Rakai, Uganda. The government of Uganda was aware of this possibility as early as 1988, when it advised, in what may be its earliest booklet on AIDS prevention, "Condoms give people a false idea they are totally safe from AIDS. The best way to avoid AIDS is to avoid causal sex and to stick to a faithful partner."[43]

There is nothing in OGAC guidance documents that discourages or restricts the promotion of condoms to adults in a generalized population. OGAC guidance does suggest that condom promotion be targeted to high-risk groups, following Uganda's successful approach during the 1990s.[44] This is for the simple fact that such groups are more likely to use condoms. In addition, promoting condoms to those who engage in high-risk

---

[41] Kajubi et al., 2005.

[42] Risk compensation and disinhibition refer to the tendency for a perception of reduced risk to make risk-taking more attractive. People may take greater risks in response to the increased sense of personal safety that comes with protective behaviors such as wearing a seatbelt or using a condom.

[43] Government of Uganda, National Resistance Movement Secretariat. *Control of AIDS: Action for Survival.* Kampala, Uganda, 1988, p. 33.

[44] There have been many recent charges that U.S. pressure has led to a current situation in which Uganda is promoting "abstinence only" to the exclusion of condoms. (For instance, *AIDS in Uganda: The Human-Rights Dimension*, Human Rights Watch, 2005, and *The Lancet*, 18 June 2005.) Yet, the broad trend over the past decade—seemingly because of pressure from foreign donors—has been far more emphasis on condom promotion at the expense of AB programs. This can be seen in Ugandan government documents such as: *The National Strategic Framework for HIV/AIDS; The National Monitoring & Evaluation Framework for HIV/AIDS Activities in Uganda 2003/04–2005/06;* and *The National Condom Policy and Strategy*, which have few references to abstinence or faithfulness. Earlier Ugandan government documents of this sort emphasized AB interventions, especially in the period 1987–89.

behaviors is also strategic in that they are more likely to be the "core transmitters" within a population.

If we follow available evidence, it appears that the actual market for condoms is very low in Africa. As observed recently in *The Lancet*, "African men and women often have more than one—typically two or perhaps three—concurrent partnerships that can overlap for months or years. This pattern differs from that of the serial monogamy more common in the west, or the one-off casual and commercial sexual encounters that occur everywhere." [45] (It should be noted that although concurrent partnerships may be more common in Africa than in the West, in any given year most Africans do not have multiple partners, concurrent or otherwise.) A pattern of concurrent partners unfortunately facilitates HIV transmission far more than serial monogamy. Making the situation worse is the fact that most men (in Africa and elsewhere) rarely use condoms with their wives or other long-term, regular partners. Years of experience in condom promotion suggest that this is unlikely to change easily or at all.

On the other hand, there is evidence that sex workers and their clients, truck drivers, soldiers posted far from home, and others are quite likely to use condoms in one-time ("one-off") or infrequent or risky sex. Such one-time sexual experiences are comparatively rare and do not add up to a substantial market for condoms. (For example, only 1.6% of Ugandan men reported paying for sex during the last year, according to the last DHS.) "Demand" for condoms is simply low in Africa and, indeed, throughout the developing world. A Population Services International survey that analyzed data from six African countries concluded that the main reasons for not using condoms have to do with poor demand. [46] Condom social marketers who

---

[45] Halperin D, Epstein H. Concurrent Sexual Partnerships Help to Explain Africa's High HIV Prevalence: Implications for Prevention. *The Lancet* 2004; 363: 4–6.

[46] Longfield et al., 2001.

have worked in Africa (including the first author) have faced this very real obstacle.

6. Does providing information about condoms lead to earlier or increased sexual activity among youth?

According to the consensus statement in *The Lancet* referred to above,[47] the priority for young people who have not yet started sexual activity should be to encourage abstinence or delay of sexual onset. For young people who have started sexual activity, returning to abstinence or being mutually faithful with an uninfected partner are the most effective ways of avoiding infection. For those young people who are sexually active and not faithful to a single uninfected partner, correct and consistent condom use should be supported.

Many sex and HIV education programs for youth in sub-Saharan Africa and other developing countries emphasize abstinence as the best means to avoid infection with HIV, but also provide factual information about condoms. This indeed is what Uganda did in its pioneer School Health Education Program that began in 1987. Because such programs encourage condom use for young people who are sexually active, they are sometimes criticized for encouraging sexual activity among youth or providing "mixed messages" to youth. Some parents and communities may object to youth receiving information about condoms. However, DHS data suggest that the majority of adults in sub-Saharan African countries agree that youth should be taught about using a condom to avoid HIV/AIDS, although a significant minority of adults do not. In most countries, approximately two-thirds of adults agree that young people aged 12 to 14 years

---

[47] Halperin, Steiner et al., 2004.

should be taught about using condoms to avoid AIDS. [48] A notable exception is Nigeria, where only 39% of adults agree that young people should receive condom education.

Table 2: Adult Support of Education on Condom Use for Youth in Sub-Saharan Africa

Country and year	Percent of adults ages 18-49 who agree that young people aged 12-14 years should be taught about using condoms to avoid AIDS	
	MALE	FEMALE
Burkina Faso 2003	71	-
Cameroon 2004	71	59
Ghana 2003	64	59
Kenya 2003	64	59
Mali 2001	65	63
Mozambique 2003	63	62
Namibia 2000	81	81
Nigeria 2003	43	36
Rwanda 2000	72	67
Tanzania 2003/4[49]	69	61
Uganda 2000/1	59	65
Zambia 2001/2	67	56
Average (unweighted)	*66*	*61*

Source: all data from DHS unless otherwise noted

Sex and HIV education programs can delay sexual onset and increase abstinence, as well as lead to greater condom use among sexually active youth. A meta-analysis by Kirby et al. found that such programs that included information on condoms while emphasizing abstinence did not lead to earlier or more frequent

---

[48] Note that the DHS question is, "Should children age 12–14 be taught about condoms to avoid AIDS?" This might be a leading question, because the wording suggests to interviewees that teaching about condoms results in avoiding AIDS, and parents may not want to seem to be disagreeing with a statement about their children avoiding AIDS.

[49] Tanzania Reproductive and Child Health Survey, 1999. Available at www.measuredhs.com.

sexual activity.[50] This meta-analysis examined the impact of school and community-based sex and HIV education programs, and included 18 studies from developing countries, and nine from Africa. All of the programs in developing countries included some information on condoms. Although approximately half of the developing country programs had no effect on delay of sexual debut, frequency of sex, or number of sexual partners, about half of the programs impacted these behaviors positively. No developing country programs led to earlier sexual debut or greater sexual activity. Yet other data from developing and developed countries have found that youth may overestimate the effectiveness of condoms, believing them to be 100% effective, and that this belief may be correlated with a lower age of sexual debut.[51] A 2002 study conducted in Uganda found that 53% of secondary school students in Kampala and 71% of 14 to 16 year old students in the rural district of Kasese believed condoms to be 100% effective against HIV infection.[52]

Whereas comprehensive programs which include accurate information on condom effectiveness can impact youth behavior positively, other data from Africa show that higher levels of condom awareness among youth do not lead to reduced risk of HIV. DHS findings among adolescents in sub-Saharan Africa found no relationship between levels of contraceptive awareness in general, or condom awareness in the context of AIDS (as measured by a correct answer to the question, "Do condoms prevent AIDS?") and either HIV seroprevalence levels or success in seroprevalence stabilization.[53] If anything, there is an inverse rela-

[50] Kirby D, Laris BA, Rolleri L. *Impact of Sex and HIV Curriculum-Based Education Programs in Schools and Communities on Sexual Behaviors of Youth. Youth Research Working Paper No. 2.* FHI/YouthNet: Arlington, VA, 2005.

[51] Grzelak S. *Teen STAR Program Evaluation in Three Countries: Poland, Chile, and USA (2002-2004).* Washington, DC: Natural Family Planning Center of Washington, DC, 2004 (unpublished).

[52] Szymon Grzelak, personal communication, 7 June 2006.

[53] Mahy M, Gupta N. *Trends and Differentials in Adolescent Reproductive Behavior in Sub-Saharan Africa.* DHS Analytical Studies No.3. Calverton, MD: Macro International and MEASURE DHS Project, 2002. Cited in Green, 2003.

tionship. The countries with the highest levels of adolescent awareness are Zimbabwe, Kenya, and Côte d'Ivoire, which all have high HIV infection rates relative to other countries in their respective regions. In fact, the condom measure is really one of *belief* in condom efficacy for AIDS prevention. Those countries in which belief among young women in condom efficacy is lowest (Senegal, Mali, Burkina Faso, Ghana) stand out as countries of low HIV seroprevalence.[54]

7. Does the ABC approach demand an unrealistic standard of behavior?

Critics of the ABC approach often make statements such as: "The behavioral bias of the ABC approach is based on the assumption that individuals all have an innate and equal power to make perfectly correct decisions about every issue in their sexual and reproductive health lives,"[55] or, "We all know that abstinence and couples being mutually faithful would be great if they were applicable to everybody's lives, but they're not."[56] Critics of ABC may argue that African culture is polygamous, that Africans have numerous partners, or that Africans start to engage in sex at an early age. According to this logic, A and B behaviors are not realistic, and risk-reduction programs are justified by the alleged reality that Africans have many sexual partners and that women in particular can do nothing about it. Many international health organizations have therefore put the majority of their prevention resources into risk reduction measures, primarily condom promotion.

Many factors can limit or take away a person's ability to practice abstinence, faithfulness, or consistent condom use.

---

[54] Green, 2003.

[55] Osborne K. The ABCs of HIV: It's Not That Simple. *AIDSLink*; 82, 1 Nov 2003.

[56] Cohen J. Prevention Cocktails: Combining Tools to Stop HIV's Spread. *Science* 2005; 309(5737): 1002–1005.

These factors can include poverty, illiteracy, instability and displacement, and gender disparity. Is an ABC approach still an effective strategy in such circumstances? In fact, some of the strongest evidence for an ABC approach comes from situations in which there were high levels of poverty, illiteracy, and instability. When Uganda began to respond to HIV/AIDS in the late 1980s and early 1990s, it was just emerging from two decades of war and extreme civil unrest. Far from being passive victims of forces beyond their control, Ugandans mounted an effective response to HIV/AIDS in spite of the difficult situations in which they were living.

Furthermore, the best biological and survey data show that for the majority of Africans, abstinence and faithfulness are not unrealistic behaviors. DHS and other survey data show that the great majority of African women and men are already practicing B and A behaviors, in that order (Tables 3 and 4). Only 3% of African women (and 23% of African men) reported multiple sexual partners in the previous year, and this figure has been quietly decreasing in recent years, beneath the "radar screen" of public discourse about global AIDS.[57] The number of Africans who practice abstinence or faithfulness in any given year is far greater than the number of Africans who practice consistent condom use. By citing these figures, we are *not* saying we should shift attention and resources away from risk reduction programs for those at high risk. We are suggesting that donors and international health organizations reconsider which behaviors are realistic and which interventions are appropriate for most Africans.

The trend in Africa is toward higher levels of monogamy, fidelity, and abstinence,[58] and the trend in HIV prevalence is incrementally downward. According to UNAIDS, at the end of

---

[57] Mahy & Gupta, 2003. Also see DHS surveys over past decade, available at www.measuredhs.com.

[58] Green, 2003.

2006 sub-Saharan Africa now had an average adult HIV prevalence rate of 5.9%, down from 6.0% in 2004.[59] This means that more than 94% of Africans ages 15 to 49 are *not* HIV infected. These welcome trends have come about in spite of the paucity or complete absence of national programs aimed at promoting fidelity and abstinence. The United States is the first major donor to fund such programs.

In the few countries where abstinence and fidelity have been promoted at the national level and backed by resources, sexual behavior has changed and rates of HIV and other STIs have decreased. Examples include Uganda, Senegal, Jamaica, Thailand, Zambia in the 1990s, Dominican Republic (after the mid-1990s), and Kenya (after the late 1990s). Data show that abstinence and faithfulness are realistic behaviors for most Africans (see Tables 3 and 4). More than half of African youth aged 15 to 19 years report abstaining from premarital sex in the previous year, according to DHS data. For example, among unmarried youth 15 to 24, 70% of Zambian youth and 71% of Ugandan youth had no sex partner in the previous year, and in some countries an even higher proportion reported abstinence. Most sexually active adults, whether married or not, report having only one partner in the previous year. In Uganda, this figure was 93%, whereas in Zambia it was 89%.[60]

---

[59] UNAIDS, 2006.
[60] DHS. Available at www.measuredhs.com.

Table 3: Premarital Sex among Youth Ages 15 to 24 in Sub-Saharan Africa

Country and year	Percent of youth ages 15-24 reporting premarital sex in last year	
	MALE	FEMALE
Benin 2001	53	44
Botswana 2001[60]	39	42
Burkina Faso 2003	32	26
Cameroon 2004	45	34
Central African Republic 1994/5	58	41
Cote d'Ivoire 1998	61	56
Eritrea 1995	10	1
Ethiopia 2000	16	2
Ghana 2003	24	30
Guinea 1999	52	27
Kenya 2003	41	21
Malawi 2000	49	27
Mali 2001	36	29
Mozambique 2003	67	54
Namibia 2000	59	46
Nigeria 2003	29	32
Rwanda 2000	9	4
Tanzania 1999[61]	57	39
Togo 1998	46	53
Uganda 2000/01	31	27
Zambia 2003[62]	33	28
Zimbabwe 1999	34	15
Average (unweighted)	*40*	*31*

Source: all data from DHS unless otherwise noted

---

[61] Botswana AIDS Impact Survey (BAIS), 2001. Available at www.measuredhs.com.

[62] Tanzania Reproductive and Child Health Survey, 1999. Available at www.measuredhs.com.

[63] Zambia Sexual Behavior Survey, 2003. Available at www.measuredhs.com.

Table 4: Multiple Partnerships in Sub-Saharan Africa

Country and survey date	Percent of sexually active adults ages 15-49 reporting multiple partners in last year	
	MALE	FEMALE
Benin 2001	28	2
Burkina Faso 2003	23	1
Cameroon 2004	40	8
Cote d'Ivoire 1998	42	6
Ethiopia 2000	11	2
Ghana 2003	15	2
Kenya 2003	17	1
Mali 2001	23	6
Mozambique 2003	35	3
Namibia 2000	22	2
Nigeria 2003	22	1
Rwanda 2000	4	6
Tanzania 2003/4[63]	27	2
Uganda 2000/01	25	3
Zambia 2001/2	27	3
Average (unweighted)	**24**	**3**

Source: all data from DHS unless otherwise noted

Condom adoption is sometimes assumed to be a simpler behavior change to adopt than that of abstinence or faithfulness. Yet condom use, especially correct and consistent condom use, is also a difficult and demanding behavior change. Condom use also depends on supply, which can be sporadic and inconsistent in many parts of the developing world. After more than 20 years of condom promotion in the developing world, levels of consistent use remain low. In no African country have consistent condom usage rates higher than 5% ever been reported, among regular sexual partners, according to an estimate from Norman Hearst.[65]

---

[64] Tanzania HIV/AIDS Indicator Survey, 2003/4. Available at www.measuredhs.com.
[65] Norman Hearst, personal communication, 16 June 2005.

8. Is the ABC approach unrealistic for women?

The argument is often made that women do not have the choice to abstain or practice faithfulness. It is a tragic fact that some women who have practiced premarital abstinence and marital fidelity have become infected by unfaithful spouses or partners. Women may be victims of rape and sexual violence, including violence within marriage, and may be made vulnerable by poverty or other circumstances. Condoms are often proposed as the solution for these women, and the ABC approach supports condom use for those at risk of HIV transmission. But condom use can be difficult if not impossible to negotiate for a woman in a coercive situation. As for married people, or others in regular sexual relationships, empirical data and anecdotal evidence show that condoms are rarely used by married couples or other regular partners. [66]

Yet African women exercise more freedom of individual choice than is often attributed to them. Last year, two-thirds of unmarried girls and women in Africa (ages 15 to 24) practiced abstinence (Table 3). Between 75% and 92% of Ugandan women say that a woman is justified in refusing sex, or sex without a condom, for reasons such as suspecting that their husband has an STI or is unfaithful, according to the DHS. Although this is a greater percentage than in many other African countries,[67] most women in other countries also report that they have the power to refuse sex with their husbands. For instance, 73% of women in Malawi, 87% in Rwanda, 82% in Tanzania, and 71% in Zimbabwe said that they could refuse sex with their husbands if they knew their husbands had STIs.[68] Yet even in countries in which a great majority of women report that a woman is justified in refusing

---

[66] Gray RH, Wawer MJ, Brookmeyer R et al. Probability of HIV-1 Transmission Per Coital Act in Monogamous, Heterosexual, HIV-1-Discordant Couples in Rakai, Uganda. *The Lancet* 2001; 357: 1149–1153.

[67] Green, 2003, pp. 171–172.

[68] Murphy et al., 2006.

sex with her husband, other data point to women's continued vulnerability. According to DHS data, a significant minority of women in Africa agree that a husband is justified in hitting or beating his wife for reasons such as burning the food, arguing with him, or refusing to have sex with him. Over half of women in Rwanda and Uganda believe that a husband is justified in hitting or beating his wife if she neglects the children.[69]

What is the solution for women who seemingly lack the power to refuse unwanted—and often risky—sex? Much attention has been given to developing products that women can control, but female condoms cannot be used without the male partner's knowledge, and a safe and effective vaginal microbicide is yet to be developed. Women who do not have the power to say no to unwanted sex probably do not have the power to insist on condom use. The best solution is for more men to be faithful and more women to be empowered to be able to refuse sex (or refuse sex without a condom). That is, the B of ABC is urgently needed, and the ABC approach must go hand in hand with addressing gender inequity. The B message must also address cross-generational sex, including rape and seduction of minor girls by older men. Under PEPFAR, prevention includes not only the promotion of ABC behaviors, but "reducing sexual violence and coercion, including child marriage, widow inheritance, and polygamy."[70] Finally, there must be consciousness raising among women and girls so that they realize and exercise the control that they do have over their sexual lives.

Uganda provides evidence that far from being insensitive to the needs and status of women, an ABC approach can go hand in hand with raising the status of women and the social responsibility of men. Under Uganda's ABC approach, women were empowered to leave husbands and boyfriends who were unfaith-

[69] DHS. Available at www.measuredhs.com.

[70] United States Leadership Against HIV/AIDS, Tuberculosis, and Malaria Act of 2003 (HR1298). Available at http://www.house.gov/pence/rsc/doc/rights%20under%20HIV-AIDS%20law.pdf (accessed 17 Mar 2006).

ful and were putting them at risk for infection. More women became economically independent,[71] and more women and girls went further in their education. Uganda also targeted men and boys with abstinence and "zero grazing" messages. Reaching men with AB messages is crucial to achieving behavior change, given prevailing power disparities between genders.

The official guidance provided by the Office of the Global AIDS Coordinator calls for communities to mobilize to reduce the vulnerability of women:

> Communities must mobilize to address the norms, attitudes, values, and behaviors that increase vulnerability to HIV, including the acceptance or tolerance of multiple casual sex partnerships, cross-generational and transactional sex, forced sex, the unequal status of women, and the sexual coercion and exploitation of young people. To stimulate such mobilization, there is an urgent need to help communities identify the ways in which they contribute to establishing and reinforcing norms that contribute to risk, vulnerability, and stigma, and to help communities identify interventions that can change norms, attitudes, values, and behaviors that increase vulnerability to HIV.[72]

Recent congressional testimony by Dr. Kent Hill, Director of USAID's Global Health Bureau, also emphasized the critical links between gender equality and HIV prevention:

> It should be noted that one way to raise the quality of the discussion of ABC prevention interventions is to insist that it take place in the context of gender issues. After all, many of the problems associated with the spread of HIV are intimately connected with the absence of gender equality, the presence of gender-based-violence and coercion typical of transactional and transgenerational sex. For all too many young girls, abstinence is not about being morally conservative, but about hav-

---

[71] Murphy et al., 2006.
[72] Office of the United States Global AIDS Coordinator for AIDS Relief, 2005.

ing the "right" to abstain. The double-standards of men who are not faithful while their wives are is a gender equity issue. In short, AB interventions must be seen as fundamentally linked to gender inequality issues.[73]

9. Does the ABC approach consider local realities such as gender and social inequalities, poverty, and cultural impediments to behavior change?

An ABC approach focuses on what individuals can do to change (or maintain) behavior, and thereby avoid or reduce risk of infection, while also recognizing that not all individuals have control over their sexual behavior. An ABCplus approach incorporates broader goals such as advancing women, increasing access to education, and decreasing poverty. Individual behavioral approaches to the prevention of sexual transmission of HIV should be complemented by larger community and societal responses, whenever possible. In countries such as Uganda where an ABC approach has been successful, broader goals such as advancing women, increasing access to education, and decreasing poverty were also pursued. These broader social changes should be pursued in addition to—and not instead of—an ABC approach that addresses individual behavior. Policy-oriented HIV strategies may pursue social goals through political leaders, legislative bodies, and action at the level of civil society and communities. Yet, most AIDS programs have a limited ability to effect broad social changes, given their limited timeframes and the range of activities that can be funded under such programs. Furthermore, although HIV prevention efforts may be strengthened by positive social changes, they are effective only when sexual behavior is changed.

---

[73] Testimony before the Subcommittee on National Security, Emerging Threats, and International Relations, Committee on Government Reform, United States House of Representatives. Washington, DC, 6 Sept, 2006.

In Uganda and in other countries, HIV prevention has been successful even though broader societal goals such as gender equality, political stability, and poverty alleviation have not been fully met. Rwanda provides a striking example. Many experts assume that strife, civil war, genocide, and breakdown of law and order—in short, social instability—would both limit AB behaviors and predict a high HIV seroprevalence rate due to increased opportunities for casual and coerced sex. Nevertheless, DHS and surveillance data from Rwanda provide powerful evidence that social instability may, in fact, have less impact than is widely assumed. A DHS population-based study recently found that Rwanda has a 3% national HIV prevalence, significantly lower than Uganda at present, and much lower than earlier UNAIDS estimates, which ran as high as 30%. In addition, recent evidence suggests that there may have been a decline in HIV prevalence in urban areas between 1998 and 2003 that was associated with low numbers of sexual partners and late sexual debut.[74]

The data in Tables 3 and 4 show that Rwanda stands out in high level of protective A and B behaviors. Only 9% of males and 4% of females ages 15 to 24 report premarital sex in the past year. Likewise, only 4% of males and 1% of females of those sexually active, ages 15 to 49, report multiple partners in the past year. Could other factors such as circumcision and condom use be responsible for low infection rates? In fact, male circumcision is not practiced widely in Rwanda and condom use, as shown in Table 1, is among the lowest in Africa. Among sexually active adults ages 15 to 49, 6% of males and 1% of females report condom use at last intercourse with any type of partner. There seems to be no readily apparent explanation other than AB behaviors to explain why an impoverished east African population that has suffered great social instability should have an HIV prevalence rate of only 3%, less than half that of Uganda's rate at present.

---

[74] Kayirangwa E, Hanson J, Munyakazi L, Kabeja A. Current Trends in Rwanda's HIV/AIDS Epidemic. *Sexually Transmitted Infections* 2006; 82(suppl_1): i27-i31.

10. Is the ABC approach overly simplistic?

The argument is sometimes made that we need to go "beyond ABC," as an ABC approach is simplistic or reductionist. Shouldn't we be doing everything to prevent AIDS: A, B, C, D (for Drugs, or De-stigmatizing AIDS), E (for Equal opportunity)...all the way to Z?

In this discussion, it is useful to distinguish between the direct and indirect factors that determine sexually transmitted HIV infection. The former (or "proximate determinants") have to do with sexual intercourse itself. The indirect factors include things like increased access to VCT and treatment for HIV and other STIs, diminishing AIDS-related stigma, poverty alleviation, effective political leadership, open discussion about sexual behavior, and educating women and improving their status. These interventions should be promoted vigorously both because they are critical matters of justice and human rights and because they likely create an environment that encourages positive changes in sexual behavior. Yet they do not in themselves directly prevent the sexual transmission of HIV. For example, creating laws that protect women from sexual exploitation may be a critical measure, but it is only when sexual behavior changes as a result that HIV transmission is directly impacted. It is widely assumed as a matter of faith that these complementary measures have the direct impact desired, yet it is important to observe empirically which measures are effective (i.e., lead directly to measurable impact), and through what mechanisms and to what extent.

The ABC approach is very likely to be more effective when undertaken in conjunction with these complementary efforts. For example, STI treatment or male circumcision can reduce the efficiency of HIV transmission. Likewise, education and economic independence of women can reduce the economic pressure to engage in commercial sex that some women experience. Such measures as widespread STI treatment and poverty alleviation are often cited as critical solutions to the HIV crisis. Although both measures undoubtedly contribute to human health and dignity and may be protective on an individual level, it is sobering to note that the evidence at a population level is somewhat more ambiguous. Data show that expanding access to VCT does not necessarily reduce HIV prevalence in a population.[75,76,77,78] Furthermore, in some countries HIV prevalence rises—rather than falls—with income level.[79] These realities should raise questions about the true relationship between many presumed HIV preventive measures and the transmission of HIV itself. The sexual transmission of HIV can be directly prevented in three basic ways: by avoiding the exposure to risk through sexual abstinence, by reducing the risk of exposure through partner faithfulness and reduction in partners, or by blocking the efficiency of transmission through a measure such as condom usage.[80] In other words, by practicing A, B, or C.[81]

Incidence and Prevalence

Throughout this document prevalence data are often cited, since with few exceptions incidence data are unavailable. Incidence—the number of *new* infections

---

[75] Matovu et al., 2003.

[76] Weinhardt et al., 1999.

[77] Wolitski et al., 1997.

[78] Glick, 2005.

[79] Shelton JD, Cassell MM, Adetunji J. Is Poverty Or Wealth at the Root of HIV? *The Lancet* 2005; 366: 1057–1058.

[80] Although condom usage can reduce transmission efficiency in the short term, other measures such as male circumcision and STI treatment can also reduce transmission efficiency in the long term.

[81] Ahmed S, Mosley H. *ABCDE...Zero HIV/AIDS*. Presentation at the Presidential Advisory Committee on HIV/AIDS, Washington, DC, 4 Aug 2003.

within a population—is of course a better measure of HIV trends than prevalence, the proportion of a population that is infected at a given time. When incidence data are unavailable, trends in prevalence among cohorts (especially 15-19, or 15-24, the group whose infections, on average, are most recent) can serve as a proxy for trends in incidence, although prevalence always lags a few years behind incidence, and can be affected by other factors.

Dr. Norman Hearst offers the following explanation of the relationship between prevalence and incidence. For prevalence to fall, the numerator of infected people must fall. (In theory, prevalence could also fall due to a big increase in the denominator, such as massive in-migration of HIV-negative people, but there may not be any real-world examples of this.) The numerator of infected people can fall in at least three ways: infected people can die, migrate away, or graduate out of the specific age-group being examined and be replaced by people who are not infected. It would take at least a few years for infected people to die in sufficient numbers to substantially lower prevalence. In fact, it might take as long as 10 years or more to reach a new steady state of prevalence after an incidence drop, since many people now live longer due to ART.

It is among the youngest age groups that changes in incidence will most quickly be reflected in changes in prevalence. Among 30 to 35-year-olds, prevalence in the new 30-year-olds entering the group is likely to already be quite high and to be similar to the prevalence of the former 35-year-olds who graduate, so the prevalence of the whole group will likely change little. For 15 to 19-year olds, changes in incidence are likely to have a substantial effect on prevalence as new 15-year-olds entering the cohort have a very low prevalence. If prevalence in 15-year-olds is almost 0, then prevalence among 15 to 19-year-olds could fall by as much as 20% of the previous level per year.

Following a substantial drop in incidence, we would expect noticeable drops in prevalence within approximately 2 years in the 15 to 19-year-old age group, within 3 to 4 years in the 15 to 24-year-old age group, and 4 or more years in older groups (longer with high ART coverage). Of course, a smaller drop in incidence might take even longer to detect by watching prevalence. This seems to match fairly well what was seen in Uganda, with incidence falling sharply in the late 1980s and notable prevalence drops starting a few years later, reaching a more-or-less steady state by the mid-1990s.[82]

We might find political leadership, open discussion of HIV/AIDS, or other factors conducive to fighting AIDS, yet no decline in HIV transmission within a country. Uganda was unique in its clear focus on what individuals themselves could do to change or maintain behavior. Uganda had strong political leadership, pioneered approaches toward reducing stigma, and brought discussion of sexual behavior out into the open. Uganda also involved HIV-infected people in public education, persuaded individuals and couples to be tested and counseled, improved the status of women, involved reli-

---

[82] Norman Hearst, personal communication, 16 June 2005.

gious organizations, enlisted traditional healers, and much more. If any country could be said to have promoted "A through Z" to prevent AIDS, it is Uganda. Yet, the message for the public was the simple one of ABC. Incorporating a range of other approaches in HIV prevention strategies can be helpful if they are designed to lead clearly to changes in sexual behavior. If they are advocated as a distraction from a strong focus on ABC-related sexual behavior changes, they are not likely to be successful.

One additional letter, or pair of letters, should be mentioned here: MC for male circumcision. An association between male circumcision and lower HIV infection rates was first noted around 1989.[83] Since then, over 40 epidemiological studies, several meta-analyses, and randomized trials in South Africa, Kenya and Uganda have investigated this association. The UNAIDS Multicentre study of four African cities found that prevalence of MC was one of the most significant factors explaining levels of HIV infection, with cities with high rates of MC having lower HIV prevalence even when sexual behavioral risk factors were similar.[84] The first randomized trial of MC, held in South Africa, found that MC has the potential to reduce HIV infection rates by 60% to 70%.[85] Subsequent randomized trials in Kenya and Uganda found that MC reduced HIV infection rates by 53% and 48%, respectively.[86] Findings to date are sufficiently strong that the U.S. Presidential Advisory Council for HIV/AIDS is recommending that the MC evidence be carefully followed, with a

---

[83] Bongaarts J, Reining P, Way P, Conant F. The Relationship between Male Circumcision and HIV Infection in African Populations. *AIDS* 1989; 3: 373–377.

[84] Auvert B, Buvé A, Lagarde E et al. Male Circumcision and HIV Infection in Four Cities in Sub-Saharan Africa. *AIDS* 2001; 15 (Suppl.): S31–40.

[85] Auvert B, Taljaard D, Lagarde E et al. Randomized, Controlled Intervention Trial of Male Circumcision for Reduction of HIV Infection Risk: The ANRS 1265 Trial. *PLoS Medicine* 2005; 2(11): 298.

[86] H.I.V. Risk Halved by Circumcision, U.S. Agency Finds. *The New York Times*, New York, 14 Dec 2006.

view toward possible policy and program recommendations, at least for generalized epidemics.[87]

11. Does the ABC approach contribute to the stigmatization and marginalization of PLWAs?

Many public health strategies promote healthy behaviors that not everyone in a population is capable of or willing to adopt. Although this may stigmatize and marginalize those who do not adopt those healthy behaviors, the benefit for those who do adopt healthy behaviors may outweigh the risks of stigmatizing some. Consider the example of smoking. Even though the best public health campaigns about the dangers of smoking may not persuade all smokers to stop smoking and may, in fact, make some smokers feel stigmatized, antismoking campaigns have been effective. It is widely believed that the health, economic, and environmental benefits of decreased smoking justify some stigmatization of those who continue to smoke. In fact, antismoking campaigns in the United States have been largely successful, and rates of lung cancer have fallen.

PLWAs are often effective leaders in the fight against HIV/AIDS. In many African countries, networks of people living with HIV/AIDS are major advocates for behavior change, including all three ABC behaviors. In the face of the HIV/AIDS crisis, advocates of an ABC approach feel that it is justified to promote an approach that has been effective in changing sexual behavior and saving lives. Some people may feel marginalized or stigmatized by an ABC approach and may face social disapproval for either engaging in or *not* engaging in A, B, or C

---

[87]   Grogan J, Smith A, Sweeney M et al. *Achieving an HIV-Free Generation: Recommendations for a New American HIV Strategy.* Washington, DC: Presidential Advisory Council for HIV/AIDS, 2005. Available at http://www.pacha.gov/pdf/PACHArev113005.pdf (accessed 2 June 2006).

behaviors. Yet, to object to the promotion of abstinence and faithfulness because some will not or cannot abstain or be faithful denies information and support to the majority of the population that does practice AB behaviors. As shown in Tables 3 and 4, in a given year, a majority of Africans already practice faithfulness (measured in not having more than one sexual partner) or abstinence.

Faith communities and leaders have been accused of contributing to stigma toward PLWAs, and some feel that it is inherently stigmatizing when faith leaders promote abstinence and faithfulness from a moral point of view. There have undoubtedly been times and situations in which faith communities and leaders have contributed to stigma. Stigma is often a problem at all levels of society, and faith communities are not immune. But in many situations, faith communities have effectively addressed stigma, encouraged compassion, and effectively promoted A and B behaviors. Uganda and Senegal stand out as African countries with relatively little AIDS-associated stigma. Both countries also promoted A and B behaviors, and partnered with Christian and Muslim faith-based organizations (FBOs) in significant ways. Rather than being seen as part of the problem, faith communities were felt to be part of the solution, and their support was enlisted at a national level.

12. Has PEPFAR imposed the ABC approach on people in the developing world?

PEPFAR has adopted an ABC approach for generalized HIV/AIDS epidemics, using Uganda's experience as a model. Some observers allege that the ABC approach is driven by the ideology of U.S. conservatives and that PEPFAR inappropriately imposed it on other countries. In fact, the ABC approach was developed and successfully implemented by Africans, without significant involvement of the United States or other large donor organizations.

Although Ugandans did not invent the ABC approach or necessarily use the term "ABC" in the beginning of the pandemic, Uganda's response was to promote abstinence, faithfulness, and later, condom use. Other countries in Africa have since adopted an ABC approach, but Uganda still provides the best example of a balanced and successful implementation of the approach.

PEPFAR has demonstrated an ability to learn from a locally developed African approach, recognizing its value in combating AIDS in the African context in particular. The success of this indigenous approach has proved once again that we should not assume that all the solutions to the problems of the poor lie outside those communities and populations, that they can be found only in the donor organizations. Africans, and particularly Ugandans, should be given the credit for developing an approach that is culturally relevant, low cost, sustainable and successful.

USAID and CDC personnel working to implement PEPFAR may resent the imposition of an approach that may be new to them, as an April 2006 United States Government Accountability Office report has noted.[88] The Congressional earmark that certain percentages be spent on AB programs can be viewed as disregard for the accumulated field experience of AIDS professionals, who believe with good reason that they understand the challenges and needs of the countries they work in far better than Washington bureaucrats. We acknowledge that it would have been much better if the need for—and value of—AB programs had emerged naturally and spontaneously through collaborative interaction between foreign advisors and African partners. We hope that if the AB spending earmarks are removed in the future, AB programs will by then have proved themselves as effective and needed primary prevention strategies, especially in Africa.

---

[88] United States Government Accountability Office. *GAO-06-395: Spending Requirement Presents Challenges for Allocating Prevention Funding under the President's Emergency Plan for AIDS Relief.* Washington, DC: GAO, April 2006.

13. Is PEPFAR promoting abstinence and faithfulness at the expense of condoms?

PEPFAR supports a comprehensive ABC approach that employs population-specific interventions that emphasize abstinence for youth and other unmarried persons, including delay of sexual debut; mutual faithfulness and partner reduction for sexually active adults; and correct and consistent use of condoms by those whose behavior places them at risk for transmitting or becoming infected with HIV. For years, there has been a standard biomedical risk reduction approach, used worldwide, that has promoted condom use, VCT, and STI treatment. Thus, a single approach using standardized program impact indicators already exists. The ABC approach incorporates the existing approach but is broader because it also promotes primary prevention, that is, A and B behaviors.

The U.S. Government is the largest single supplier of condoms worldwide, and under PEPFAR annual condom procurement has been steadily rising. The Office of the Global AIDS Coordinator estimates that in 2005 the U.S. Government shipped more than 612 million condoms to Africa, Asia, and Latin America, the greatest annual figure since 1995.[89,90] Despite this, it is often alleged that PEPFAR is promoting an "abstinence-only" strategy. This is inaccurate both because of PEPFAR's continued support of condoms for at-risk populations and because the ABC approach emphasizes fidelity as well as abstinence (and is therefore not "abstinence only").

It has also been alleged that Uganda has begun to discontinue condoms in favor of an abstinence-only strategy. [91] In 2005, a supply problem (caused by the recall of a large batch

---

[89] Donnelly J. U.S. Condom Policy in Africa Targets "High-Risk" Areas. *Boston Globe*, 8 Sept 2005.

[90] Chaya et al., 2004.

[91] Cohen J, Schleifer R, Tate T. AIDS in Uganda: The Human-Rights Dimension. *The Lancet* 2005; 365: 2075–2076.

of condoms) fueled allegations that Uganda was experiencing a severe shortage of condoms. Ugandan officials responded by saying that Uganda continues to promote all three components of the ABC approach and that Uganda had sufficient stocks of condoms. In fact, at the time of reports of critical condom shortages Uganda procured 80 million condoms.[92]

There is evidence that Uganda has been shifting away from AB messages and interventions and moving toward a greater emphasis on condom use, testing, and other medical interventions. In Uganda's current national Strategic Framework for HIV/AIDS document, which is a blueprint for all the activities supported in Uganda to combat AIDS, there are virtually no A or B elements. That is, there are no specific objectives or impact indicators related to abstinence or faithfulness. The document is mostly concerned with condoms, testing, STIs, future vaccines, future microbicides, and antiretroviral drugs. The document reflects the biomedical "products and procedures" approach to HIV prevention rather than a sociobehavioral approach. Examination of other national AIDS documents in Uganda shows the same trend.[93] A 2005 survey of AIDS-related media content in Uganda carried out by the Steadman Media Group showed that in the previous three years, most of the AIDS-related media expenditures had been for the promotion of condoms and VCT. Only about 4% of content was on abstinence.[94] Proponents of the ABC approach are concerned that Uganda may be turning away from its proven prevention strategy, possibly influenced by advice and funding from international donors.

---

[92] U.S. Harming Uganda's AIDS Battle. *BBC News*, 30 Aug 2005. Available at http://news.bbc.co.uk/2/hi/africa/ 4195968.stm (accessed 27 Nov 2005).

[93] For example, the *National Monitoring & Evaluation Framework for HIV/AIDS Activities in Uganda, 2003/04–2005/06*, and the *National Condom Policy and Strategy.*

[94] Steadman Media Group. *AIDS Information, Education and Communication: A Comparative Review Of Expenditure on ABC Abstinence, Being Faithful and Condom in the Electronic Media: A Survey Carried out by the Steadman Media Group.* 2005. Interreligious Council of Uganda, Kampala.

14. A recent study suggested that condoms and mortality from AIDS—and not abstinence and faithfulness—had caused HIV prevalence to decline in Uganda. Does this mean that an ABC approach didn't work in Uganda after all?

In February 2005, Wawer, Gray et al. presented a paper at the Conference on Retroviruses and Opportunistic Infections.[95] This paper was widely interpreted as proving that condoms and mortality from AIDS—and not abstinence and faithfulness—were responsible for Uganda's decline in HIV prevalence. Major newspapers reported on the story under such headlines as: "Uganda's HIV success has more to do with condoms than abstinence"[96]; "Uganda: Condoms outshine abstinence in Aids battle"[97]; "Uganda's decline in HIV/AIDS prevalence attributed to increased condom use"[98]; and "HIV study downplays abstinence in Uganda."[99] The UNAIDS Epidemic Update 2005 reported about Uganda, "Evidence of such [behavior] change has been uneven, with researchers observing no significant increases in abstinence or fidelity... most of the momentum for Rakai's decline in prevalence appears to have derived from higher mortality rates."[100] In citing this unpublished paper, UNAIDS overlooked or ignored findings published in leading peer-reviewed journals such as *Science*, *The Lancet*, and *British Medical Journal*, all concluding that partner reduction was the major factor in Uganda's prevalence decline.[101]

---

[95] Wawer MJ, Gray R et al. *Declines in HIV Prevalence in Uganda: Not as Simple as ABC.* Presentation at Conference on Retroviruses and Opportunistic Infections. Boston, MA, 22 Feb 2005.

[96] *The Advocate*, Los Angeles, 25 Feb 2005.

[97] *AllAfrica.com*, Africa, 24 Feb 2005.

[98] *Medical News Today*, United Kingdom, 26 Feb 2005.

[99] *Newsday*, New York, 25 Feb 2005.

[100] UNAIDS, 2005a.

[101] See Allen T, Heald S. HIV/AIDS Policy in Africa: What Has Worked in Uganda and What Has Failed in Botswana? *Journal of International Development* 2004; 16: 1141–1154; Halperin & Epstein, 2004; Stoneburner & Low-Beer, 2004; Shelton et al., 2004.

Wawer and Gray suggest that because after 1994 there were higher levels of condom use and lower levels of monogamy and abstinence in Rakai, Uganda, condom use (and mortality rates) had accounted for continuing declines in HIV prevalence. Dr. Henry Mosley makes the following points about the error of this assumption[102]:

> The Rakai study intensively covered only a small population in one district of Uganda and thus is difficult to generalize for all of Uganda. Furthermore, the period of intensive observation documenting changes in HIV incidence and prevalence and in trends in sexual abstinence and multiple partners was 1994–95 to 2002–03, well after the major decline in HIV prevalence in most of Uganda.
>
> The data do permit the following two major conclusions regarding the effects of ABC on HIV trends in this district.
>
> 1) Over the entire study period A, B, and C did change as follows: men 15–19 reporting sexual abstinence *declined* from 60% to 47%; men 15 to 49 reporting 1 or more non-marital partners *increased* from 35% to 44%; men 15–49 reporting consistent condom use with last non-marital sexual partner *increased* from 18% to 73%. (Similar trends in ABC were seen among women.) The net effect of these countervailing trends was essentially *no change* in the annual incidence of HIV. Thus there is no evidence that condom use has altered the course of the epidemic during the study period. Rather the compensating effects of changes in A, B and C have kept the incidence stable.
>
> 2) Epidemiologically, it can be shown that most of the decline in prevalence during the study period must come from a *decline in incident cases 7 to 8 years earlier,* not from a rise in death rates as reported by the authors. This analysis estimates that incident cases in the period 1987 to 1995 must have declined by about 40%. This was a period when condom use must have been well below the 18% for

---

[102] Mosley, 2005.

men and 8% from women reported in 1994–95. The only factors reasonably accounting for this dramatic decline in this early period must have been and increase in A and B behaviors.

The countervailing trends in A, B, and C behaviors suggest that what is being observed with increasing condom use is "behavioral disinhibition." Other protective behaviors are being discarded as condoms are being adopted. This could be an explanation for why condom programs alone have not been associated with any amelioration of population-wide heterosexual AIDS epidemics in many sub-Saharan African countries.

A multi-country analysis which used mathematical modeling to assess the effects of mortality and sexual behavior change on HIV prevalence also concluded that in Uganda, HIV prevalence has declined further than would be expected from the effects of mortality alone.[103]

15. Even if the ABC approach did work in Uganda, is there evidence that it could work in other countries?

The ABC approach has been implemented to varying degrees in Senegal, Jamaica, Zambia, Kenya, and among Thailand's general population, and elsewhere, with varying degrees of positive results in at least the countries just named.[104] In Zambia, there were significant declines in HIV among youth in the 1990s,[105] but this was not sustained after about 1998. In Zimbabwe and Kenya, there have been recent A and B behavior changes associated with a decline in HIV prevalence.

---

[103] Hallett TB, Aberle-Grasse J, Bello G et al. Declines in HIV Prevalence Can Be Associated with Changing Sexual Behavior in Uganda, Urban Kenya, Zimbabwe, and Urban Haiti. *Sexually Transmitted Infections* 2006; 82(suppl_1): i1-i8.
[104] Green, 2003.
[105] Bessinger et al., 2003.

Kenya provides a recent example of a successful ABC approach. In Kenya, the major response to AIDS before 1999 was condom supply and promotion. There was little or no impact on the pandemic. Finally, the Kenyan government implemented an ABC approach. In addition, faith-based groups were mobilized. AIDS education was implemented in schools. Educators and officials emphasized the seriousness of the epidemic, and government officials were told that they must mention AIDS every time they had a public meeting.

As illustrated in Figure 5, which compares Kenya DHS data from 1998 and 2003, there was little change in condom use, especially among men. There was a significant increase in the proportion of unmarried people reporting no sex in the past year, and a roughly 50% decline in the proportion of men and women reporting more than two partners in the past year.

Figure 5: ABC Behaviors in Kenya, 1998 to 2003

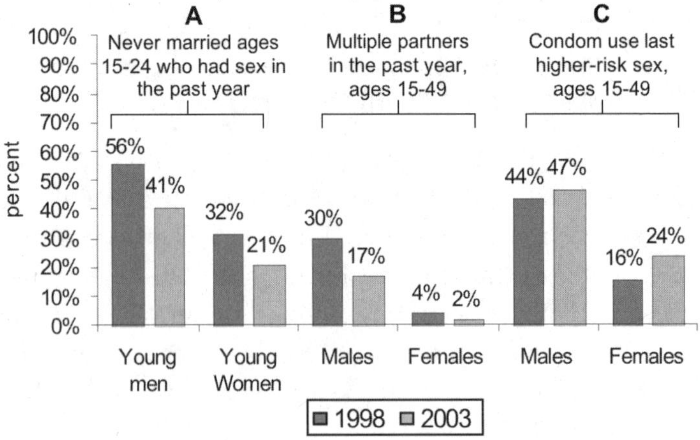

Source: Demographic Health Surveys

What impact did this have? Comparisons between population-based and antenatal clinic (ANC) surveys, using sophisticated statistical techniques, "suggest that the epidemic in Kenya peaked in the late 1990s with an overall prevalence of 10% in adults, and declined to 7% by 2003."[106] The B component again appears to be the crucial factor associated with national HIV prevalence decline, just as in Uganda. Those reporting two or more partners in the past year in the 2003 DHS were twice as likely to be HIV infected as those reporting one partner. National prevalence is now slightly lower than that of Uganda, which is estimated at 7% using the same population-based method. The fact that 80% of Kenyan men are circumcised likely contributes to lower infections rates in Kenya.

There are also countries like Zimbabwe where A and B interventions seem not to be much emphasized outside of faith-based organizations. Yet, in Zimbabwe, we see A and B behavior changes, and, as in Uganda and Kenya, they seem to be the primary factors associated with HIV prevalence decline. A study in Manicaland in rural eastern Zimbabwe examined these factors as well as possible confounders such as mortality and migration rates. This study found that between 1998 and 2003 there was a decrease in overall adult HIV prevalence (from 23.0% to 20.5%), with steeper reductions of 23% and 49% in young men and women. During this same period, there was an increase in AB behaviors. For instance, the percentage of 17 to 19-year-old men who reported having started sex decreased from 45% to 27%, and the percentage of men who reported having a casual partner in the last month decreased from 26% to 13%.[107]

Similar trends in declining HIV prevalence have been seen in recent national surveillance data from ANCs in

---

[106] UNAIDS, 2005a.
[107] Gregson S, Garnett GP, Nyamukapa CA, et al. HIV Decline Associated with Behavior Change in Eastern Zimbabwe. *Science* 3 Feb 2006; 311: 664–666.

Zimbabwe.[108] ANC data showed a decline in HIV prevalence among pregnant women from 32.1% in 2000 to 23.9% in 2004.[109] A 2005 UNAIDS study that evaluated multiple sources of data also concluded that HIV prevalence had fallen in Zimbabwe over the previous five years. In addition, this study stated that B behaviors—reductions in rates of sexual partner change—contributed to declines in HIV incidence.[110] This study also credited high rates of condom use with nonregular partners, which were already high by 1999.

The data from Zimbabwe are strikingly similar to those of Kenya, shown above. In Zimbabwe, as in Kenya, there were increases in AB behaviors between 1998 and 2003, and little change in condom use over this time period. Ambassador Mark Dybul, U.S. Global AIDS Coordinator, observed about the evidence from Zimbabwe: "Perhaps one of the most interesting things is that the greatest behaviour change was in abstinence and fidelity. The relative change in condom use was not as remarkable."[111] Gregson, the primary author of the study in Manicaland, remarked that "it is important to note that all three types of behavior change seem important in Zimbabwe. We need to be promoting all the different prevention possibilities."[112]

These findings from Kenya and Zimbabwe are corroborated by a multi-country analysis that sought to determine through mathematical modeling whether declines in HIV prevalence in

[108] Hayes R, Weiss H. Enhanced: Understanding HIV Epidemic Trends in Africa. *Science* 3 Feb 2006; 311: 620–621.

[109] Mahomva A, Greby S, Dube S, et al. HIV prevalence and trends from data in Zimbabwe, 1997–2004. *Sexually Transmitted Infections* 2006; 82(suppl_1): i42-i47.

[110] UNAIDS. *Evidence for HIV Decline in Zimbabwe: A Comprehensive Review of the Epidemiological Data.* Geneva: UNAIDS, 2005b. Available at http://data.unaids.org/Publications/IRCpub06/Zimbabwe_Epi_report_Nov05_en.pdf (accessed 2 Mar 2006).

[111] Check E. HIV Infection in Zimbabwe Falls at Last. *BioEd Online* 2 Feb 2006. Available at http://www.bioedonline.org/news/news.cfm?art=2318 (accessed 2 Mar 2006).

[112] Check, 2006.

countries with generalized epidemics were associated with changes in sexual behavior or were simply an effect of natural epidemic patterns such as mortality. The study concluded that in Uganda, parts of Kenya, Zimbabwe, and urban Haiti, "HIV prevalence has declined further than would be expected through the effects of mortality alone." These declines in prevalence were attributed to changed sexual behavior.[113] In Haiti, prevalence has decreased since 2000 from approximately 5.5% to 3% among women ages 15 to 44. This decline in HIV prevalence was preceded by an increase in B behaviors. There was a 20% decline in the mean number of sexual partners between 1994 and 2000. In addition, there was also a two- to threefold increase in condom use between 2000/1 and 2003.[114]

When linking data on behavior change to changes in HIV prevalence, it should be remembered that prevalence is a lagging indicator of incidence, the rate of new infections. Showing changes in prevalence for two points in time and changes in behavior during those same two points in time can be misleading. The data from Haiti do show an increase in B behaviors preceding a decline in HIV prevalence. For Kenya and Zimbabwe, it would be better to look at changes in behavior somewhat earlier (e.g., between 1994 and 1999) and relate these changes to later prevalence decline.[115] Unfortunately, there is a lack of data on factors such as partner reduction or the proportion of youth 15–19 who had sexual intercourse in the previous 12 months (a better indicator of behavior change than age of sexual debut, which is sometimes used). PEPFAR's recommended indicators do include A and B behaviors and aim to increase the available data about these behaviors.

Ethiopia provides another possible example of a successful ABC approach, although the above mentioned multi-country

---

[113] Hallett et al, 2006.
[114] Hallett et al, 2006.
[115] We thank Jim Shelton of USAID for reminding us to mention this.

study concluded that although Ethiopia experienced a decline in national HIV prevalence between 2001 and 2003 (from 14% to 12%), these changes were not necessarily due to changes in sexual risk behavior.[116] Yet data from Addis Ababa showed a decline in HIV prevalence among women at ANC clinics, from 18.2% in 1997 to 11.8% in 2003. In addition, data from two VCT sites in Addis Ababa showed a decline in HIV prevalence from 29.1% in 2002 to 14.9% in 2004, for adults aged 15 to 44. There was an even greater decline for youth aged 15-24, from 22.0% in 2002 to 9.0% in 2004. Along with declines in HIV prevalence there was an associated decline in risky behaviors among VCT clients. The mean number of casual partners reported in the three months prior to testing declined among all clients between 2002 and 2004, from 1.0 to 0.6. Condom use did not increase, and in fact the proportion of clients ages 25-49 who reported never using a condom increased somewhat. Over 60% of clients reporting never using condoms consistently and fewer than 35% of clients reporting having used condoms at their last sexual inter-course.[117]

16. In mature epidemics, a large percentage of new HIV infections can occur in discordant couples. How can the ABC approach curb transmission among these couples?

Condom usage rates among married or regular partners are typically low, with less than 5% of regular partners reporting consistent use.[118] Couples' counseling may increase usage rates among discordant couples, but this usage is often imperfect (inconsistent) and the use of biological markers has shown that actual usage is

---

[116] Hallet et al, 2006.

[117] Hladik W, Shabbir I, Jelaludin A, Woldu A, Tsehaynesh M, Tadesse W. HIV/AIDS in Ethiopia: where is the epidemic heading? *Sexually Transmitted Infections* 2006; 82(suppl_1): i32-i35.

[118] Norman Hearst, personal communication, 16 June 2005.

often not as high as reported usage.[119] Serodiscordant couples report abstinence as well as condom usage as strategies to avoid infection, and research has shown that many HIV-negative females would prefer abstinence had their partners not refused.[120]

Discordant couple also clearly need the "be faithful" message. Even if every uninfected partner became infected, this would not perpetuate the epidemic unless infected people infected more than one partner. (For epidemics to be sustained, the "reproductive number" must be greater than one.) Thus, the B message, if followed, has a strong protective effect at the broader population level. Even at the individual level, sex with multiple partners can lead to superinfection,[121] making AIDS worse and complicating the prospect of treatment. Therefore, even for serodiscordant couples, A and B messages can have great relevance.

Some observers have suggested that the AB components are no longer as relevant in an era of antiretroviral treatment (ART). A recent public statement from the Ugandan government—the lead author being the official who ran Uganda's national AIDS Control program in the earliest years—is that ABC is needed even more in the era of antiretroviral treatment:

> Abstinence, being faithful, and condom use are complementary, synergistic, and inseparable components in the country's HIV/AIDS national prevention and control programmes, and we need to roll out these prevention messages with extra urgency now, in the era of ART.[122]

---

[119] Allen et al., 2003.

[120] Bunnell et al., 2005.

[121] Superinfection occurs when a person becomes infected by two different strains of the HIV virus.

[122] Okware S, Kinsman J, Onyango S et al. Revisiting the ABC Strategy: HIV Prevention in the Era of Antiretroviral Therapy. *Postgraduate Medical Journal* 2005; 81: 625. Available at http://pmj.bmjjournals.com/cgi/reprint/81/960/625 (accessed 3 Jan 2006).

Conclusion

This document presents a great deal of data on the efficacy of the A and B components of the ABC approach as they are the least understood components and for many raise the most concerns. Although major organizations and agencies working in HIV prevention have several decades of experience in designing and implementing condom programs, there is far less experience in AB programs. Prior to the adoption of the ABC approach by USAID and PEPFAR in 2002 and 2003, major AIDS organizations had not put significant resources into abstinence or faithfulness interventions anywhere in the world. There is, therefore, a shortage of experience and evidence about how best to implement AB programs, although the data presented in this paper suggest that such interventions can be highly effective in reducing HIV transmission. Yet many in the international health community continue to express concern over, and resistance to, AB interventions, alleging that they have not proven effective. As evidence accumulates that A and especially B behaviors are critical in reducing HIV transmission, particularly within generalized epidemics, one must question whether the continuing controversy is truly a debate over evidence or ideology.

There has also been resistance to, and misinformation about, condoms. This should be addressed, although condom opponents or skeptics are not normally represented in the major

AIDS and reproductive health organizations. Until quite recently, those unwilling to promote condoms, such as Catholic organizations, were simply excluded from HIV prevention programs that were funded by major donor organizations.

Recently, this bias has been changing, and major donors have come to realize that FBOs must be key partners in confronting AIDS. Some FBOs choose not to promote condoms, but other organizations undoubtedly will, and, by promoting abstinence and faithfulness, FBOs can be part of an overall balanced ABC approach. PEPFAR has been modeled on Uganda's approach, where the government made FBOs key partners as it confronted AIDS. The Ugandan government recognized, for instance, that Catholics represented nearly 40% of the population and were major providers of treatment for PLWAs and of care and support for PLWAs, orphans, and vulnerable children. Catholics were also willing and able to effectively promote the AB components of HIV prevention, and the government realized they would be less likely to oppose condom promotion if they were working collaboratively with major donors and NGOs in prevention. The Ugandan government, although not necessarily its foreign backers, also felt confident that A and B interventions were central to an effective AIDS prevention effort in Uganda, a confidence supported by later evidence.

The authors agree with the consensus statement published in *The Lancet* and endorsed by over 150 scientists, public health experts, and AIDS activists. This statement says about the ABC approach:

> All three elements of this approach are essential to reducing HIV incidence, although the emphasis placed on individual elements needs to vary according to the target population. Although the overall programmatic mix should include an appropriate balance of A, B, and C interventions, it is not essential that every organisation promote all three elements:

each can focus on the part(s) they are most comfortable supporting. However, all people should have accurate and complete information about different prevention options, including all three elements of the ABC approach.[1]

Finally, we wish to stress that we are not arguing for shifting attention and resources away from those at high risk, including the powerless, oppressed, exploited, raped, and abused. We *are* saying that it is inaccurate to characterize all people this way (or all Africans, in the context of this document), and that we can no longer target the majority of HIV prevention resources to this minority group. It is a tragedy that all-or-nothing thinking and polemics have dominated the AIDS debate to date and have deemed the only compassionate response one that targets the most oppressed and treats everyone as equally high risk. Reducing the risk of HIV infection for all people is the only truly compassionate response. What has been missing in this bitter debate is a calm, even-handed, balanced viewpoint that recognizes that some resources clearly must be targeted to high-risk groups, while some resources must be directed to what survey and epidemiological evidence show are the majority of people. To target only those at high-risk is to effectively ignore most of the population. Targeting both minority (high-risk) and majority populations need not result in diminished quality or even quantity of prevention resources going to either group. It is only catastrophist, polemical, all-or-nothing thinking that would have us believe otherwise. If Uganda, with very few resources in the early years of its response to AIDS, could design and implement a *balanced and targeted* ABC program, surely the major donors with billions of dollars can do the same.

---

[1] Halperin, Steiner et al., 2004.

References

Ahmed S, Lutalo T, Wawer M, Serwadda D, Sewankambo NK, Nalugoda F et al. HIV Incidence and Sexually Transmitted Disease Prevalence Associated with Condom Use: A Population Study in Rakai, Uganda. *AIDS* 2001; 15: 2171–2179.

Ahmed S, Mosley H. *ABCDE...Zero HIV/AIDS.* Presentation at the Presidential Advisory Committee on HIV/AIDS, Washington, DC, 4 Aug 2003.

Allen S, Meinzen-Derr J, Kautzman M et al. Sexual Behavior of HIV Discordant Couples after HIV Counseling and Testing. *AIDS* 2003; 17(5): 733–740.

Allen T, Heald S. HIV/AIDS policy in Africa: What Has Worked in Uganda and What Has Failed in Botswana? *Journal of International Development* 2004; 16: 1141–1154.

Auvert B, Taljaard D, Lagarde E, Sobngwi-Tambekou J, Sitta R, Puren A. Randomized, Controlled Intervention Trial of Male Circumcision for Reduction of HIV Infection Risk: The ANRS 1265 Trial. *PLoS Medicine* 2005; 2(11): 298.

Auvert B, Buvé A, Lagarde E, Kahindo M, Chege J, Rutenberg N et al. Male Circumcision and HIV Infection in Four Cities in Sub-Saharan Africa. *AIDS* 2001; 15(Suppl.): S31–40.

Bessinger R, Akwara P, Halperin D. *Sexual Behavior, HIV, and Fertility Trends: A Comparative Analysis of Six Countries.* Calverton, MD: ORC Macro, the Measure Project, and United States Agency for International Development. Available at www.cpc.unc.edu/measure/publications/pdf/sr-03-21b.pdf (accessed 3 Jan 2006).

Bongaarts J, Reining P, Way P, Conant F. The Relationship between Male Circumcision and HIV Infection in African Populations. *AIDS* 1999; 3: 373–377.

Botswana AIDS Impact Survey (BAIS), 2001. Available at www.measuredhs.com.

Bunnell RE, Nassozi J, Marum E, Mubangizi J, Malamba S, Dillon B, Kalule J, Bahizi J, Musoke N, Mermin JH. Living with Discordance: Knowledge, Challenges, and Prevention Strategies of HIV-Discordant Couples in Uganda. *AIDS Care* 2005; 17(8): 999–1012.

Chaya N, Amen K, Fox M. *Condoms Count: Meeting the Need in the Era of HIV/AIDS: 2004 Data Update.* 2004. Population Action International. Available at http://www.populationaction.org/resources/publications/condomscount/downloads/2004updateInsert_final.pdf (accessed 8 Apr 2006).

Check E. HIV Infection in Zimbabwe Falls at Last. *BioEd Online* 2 Feb 2006. Available at http://www.bioedonline.org/news/news.cfm?art=2318 (accessed 2 Mar 2006).

Cohen J. Prevention Cocktails: Combining Tools to Stop HIV's Spread. *Science* 2005; 309(5737): 1002–1005.

Cohen J, Schleifer R, Tate T. AIDS in Uganda: The Human-Rights Dimension. *The Lancet* 2005; 365: 2075–2076.

Cohen MS, Eron JJ. Sexual HIV Transmission and its Prevention. *Continuing Medical Education Series*; 27 June 2001. Available at http://www.medscape.com.

Demographic and Health Surveys (DHS). http://www.measuredhs.com (accessed 15 Nov 2005).

Family Health International. *AIDS Control and Prevention Project: Final Report for the AIDSCAP Program in Thailand November 1991 to September 1996.* Available at http://www.fhi.org/en/HIVAIDS/pub/Archive/aidscapreports/finalreportAIDSCAPthailand/index.htm (accessed 3 Jan 2006).

Glick P. *Scaling Up HIV Voluntary Counseling and Testing in Africa: What Can Evaluation Studies Tell Us about Potential Prevention Impacts?* Strategies and Analysis for Growth and Access (SAGA) Working Paper. Cornell University, Mar 2005.

Government of Uganda, National Resistance Movement Secretariat. *Control of AIDS: Action for Survival.* Kampala, Uganda, 1988.

Gray RH, Wawer MJ, Brookmeyer R, Sewankambo NK, Serwadda D, Wabwire-Mangen F, Lutalo T, Li X, vanCott T, Quinn TC.. Probability of HIV-1 Transmission per Coital Act in Monogamous, Heterosexual, HIV-1-Discordant Couples in Rakai, Uganda. *The Lancet* 2001; 357: 1149–1153.

Green EC. Indigenous or Western Response to African AIDS? in *Indigenous Knowledge: Local Pathways to Global Development*, Woytek R, Shroff-Mehta P, Mohan PC (eds). Washington, DC: World Bank, Africa Region Knowledge and Learning Center, 2004, pp. 18–24.

Green EC. *Rethinking AIDS Prevention.* Westport, CT: Praeger, 2003.

Green EC, Halperin DT, Nantulya V, Hogle JA. Uganda's HIV Prevention Success: The Role of Sexual Behavior Change and the National Response. *AIDS and Behavior* 2006; 10(4): 335-346.

Green EC, Nantulya V, Stoneburner R, Stover J. *What Happened in Uganda? Declining HIV Prevalence, Behavior Change, and the National Response.* Washington, DC: USAID, 2002. Available at http://www.usaid.gov/our_work/global_health/aids/Countries/africa/uganda_report.pdf (accessed 8 Apr 2006).

Gregson S, Garnett GP, Nyamukapa CA, Hallett TB, Lewis JJC, Mason PR, Chandiwana SK, Anderson RM. HIV Decline Associated with Behavior Change in Eastern Zimbabwe. *Science,* 3 Feb 2006; 311: 664–666.

Grogan, J, Smith A, Sweeney M, Mason A, Green E. *Achieving an HIV-Free Generation: Recommendations for a New American HIV Strategy.* Washington, DC: Presidential Advisory Council for HIV/AIDS, 2005. Available at http://www.pacha.gov/pdf/PACHArev113005.pdf (accessed 2 June 2006).

Grzelak S. *Teen STAR Program Evaluation in Three Countries: Poland, Chile, and USA (2002-2004).* Washington, DC: Natural Family Planning Center of Washington, DC, 2004 (unpublished).

Hallett TB, Aberle-Grasse J, Bello G, Boulos LM, Cayemittes MPA, Cheluget B, Chipeta J, Dorrington R, Dube S, Ekra AK, Gaillard EM, Garcia-Calleja JM, Garnett GP, Greby S, Gregson S, Grove JT, Hader S, Hanson J, Hladik W, Ismail S, Kassim S, Kirungi W, Kouassi L, Mahomva A, Marum L,

Maurice C, Nolan M, Rehle T, Stover J, Walker N. Declines in HIV Prevalence Can Be Associated with Changing Sexual Behavior in Uganda, Urban Kenya, Zimbabwe, and Urban Haiti. *Sexually Transmitted Infections* 2006; 82(suppl_1): i1-i8.

Halperin DT, Epstein H. Concurrent Sexual Partnerships Help to Explain Africa's High HIV Prevalence: Implications for Prevention. *The Lancet* 2004; 363: 4–6.

Halperin DT, Steiner MJ, Cassell MM, Green EC, Kirby D, Hearst N, Gayle H. The Time Has Come for Common Ground on Preventing Sexual Transmission of HIV. *The Lancet* 2004; 364: 1913–1915.

Hayes R, Weiss H. Enhanced: Understanding HIV Epidemic Trends in Africa. *Science* 3 Feb 2006; 311: 620–621.

Hearst N, Chen S. Condom Promotion for AIDS Prevention in the Developing World: Is it Working? *Studies in Family Planning* 2004; 35(1): 39–47.

Hearst N, Chen S. Condoms for AIDS Prevention in the Developing World: A Review of the Scientific Literature. Geneva: UNAIDS, 12 Jan 2003. (Submitted, but never released. Summary of report available at www.usp.br/nepaids/condom.pdf, and major findings presented in Hearst & Chen 2004.)

Hladik W, Shabbir I, Jelaludin A, Woldu A, Tsehaynesh M, Tadesse W. HIV/AIDS in Ethiopia: where is the epidemic heading? *Sexually Transmitted Infections* 2006; 82(suppl_1): i32-i35.

Hulley SB, Cummings SR, Browner WS, Grady D, Hearst N, Newman TB. *Designing Clinical Research: An Epidemiologic Approach, 2nd Edition.* Philadelphia: Lippincott, Williams & Wilkins, 2001.

Kajubi P, Kamya MR, Kamya S, Chen S, McFarland W, Hearst N. Increasing Condom Use without Reducing HIV Risk: Results of a Controlled Community Trial in Uganda. *Journal of Acquired Immune Deficiency Syndromes* 2005; 40(1): 77–82.

Kayirangwa E, Hanson J, Munyakazi L, Kabeja A. Current Trends in Rwanda's HIV/AIDS Epidemic. *Sexually Transmitted Infections* 2006; 82(suppl_1): i27-i31.

Kirby D, Laris BA, Rolleri L. Impact of Sex and HIV Curriculum-Based Education Programs in Schools and Communities on Sexual Behaviors of Youth. *Youth Research Working Paper No. 2.* Arlington, VA: FHI/YouthNet, 2005.

Longfield K, Agha S, Kusanthan T, Klein M, Berman J. *Non-Use of Condoms: What Role Do Supply, Demand, and Acceptance Play in the 'Condom Gap'?* Presentation at the International Conference on AIDS and STDs in Africa, Ouagadougou, Burkina Faso, Dec 2001.

Mahomva A, Greby S, Dube S, Mugurungi O, Hargrove J, Rosen D, Dehne KL, Gregson S, St Louis M, Hader S. HIV prevalence and trends from data in Zimbabwe, 1997–2004. *Sexually Transmitted Infections* 2006; 82(suppl_1): i42-i47.

Mahy M, Gupta N. *Trends and Differentials in Adolescent Reproductive Behavior in Sub-Saharan Africa.* DHS Analytical Studies No. 3. Calverton, MD: Macro International and MEASURE DHS Project, 2002.

Matovu JKB, Kigozi G, Nalugoda F. *Repetitive VCT, Sexual Risk Behavior and HIV-Incidence in Rakai, Uganda.* Presentation at the Uganda Virus Research Institute, Entebbe, Uganda, 28 Nov 2003.

Mekonnen Y, Sanders E, Aklilu M, Tsegayea A, Rinke de Wita TF, Schaap A, Wolday D, Geskus R, Coutinho RA, Fontaneta AL. Evidence of changes in sexual behaviours among male factory workers in Ethiopia. *AIDS* 2003, 17: 223-231.

Mosley H. Declining HIV in Uganda Cannot Be Explained by Mortality or Condoms (Letter). *British Medical Journal* 2005; 330: 496.

Murphy E, Greene ME, Duong T. *Defending the ABCs: A Feminist Perspective on AIDS Prevention.* Presentation at African Successes: Can Behavior-Based Solution Make a Crucial Contribution to HIV Prevention in Sub-Saharan Africa? Munyonyo, Uganda, 17-20 Dec 2006.

National AIDS and STI Control Programme (NASCOP), Ministry of Health, Kenya. *AIDS in Kenya: Trends, Interventions and Impact, 7th ed.* Nairobi: NASCOP, 2005.

Office of the United States Global AIDS Coordinator for AIDS Relief. *ABC Guidance for United States Government In-Country Staff and Implementing Partners Applying the ABC Approach to Preventing Sexually Transmitted HIV Infections within The President's Emergency Plan for AIDS Relief.* Washington, DC, Mar 2005.

Office of the United States Global AIDS Coordinator for AIDS Relief. *The President's Emergency Plan for AIDS Relief: U.S. Five-year Global HIV/AIDS Strategy.* Washington, DC, Feb 2004.

Okware, S, Kinsman J, Onyango S, Opio A, Kaggwa P. Revisiting the ABC Strategy: HIV Prevention in the Era of Antiretroviral Therapy. *Postgraduate Medical Journal* 2005; 81: 625. Available at http://pmj.bmjjournals.com/cgi/reprint/81/960/625 (accessed 3 Jan 2006).

Osborne K. The ABCs of HIV: It's Not That Simple. *Global AIDSLink* 2003; 82 (1 Nov 2003).

Phoolcharoen W. HIV/AIDS Prevention in Thailand: Success and Challenges. *Science* 19 June 1998; 280 (5371): 1873–1874.

Richens J, Imrie J, Copas A. Condoms and Seat Belts: The Parallels and the Lessons. *The Lancet* 2000; 29: 400.

Shelton JD, Cassell MM, Adetunji J. Is Poverty or Wealth at the Root of HIV? *The Lancet* 2005; 366: 1057–1058.

Shelton JD, Halperin DT, Nantulya V, Potts M, Gayle HD, Holmes KK. Partner Reduction is Crucial for Balanced "ABC" Approach to HIV Prevention. *British Medical Journal* 2004; 328: 891–893.

Shelton J, Johnston B. Condom Gap in Africa: Evidence from Donor Agencies and Key Informants. *British Medical Journal* 2001; 323: 139.

Steadman Media Group. *AIDS Information, Education and Communication: A Comparative Review Of Expenditure on ABC Abstinence, Being Faithful and Condom in the Electronic Media: A Survey Carried out by the Steadman Media Group.* 2005. Interreligious Council of Uganda, Kampala.

Stoneburner RL, Low-Beer D. Population-Level HIV Declines and Behavioral Risk Avoidance in Uganda. *Science* 2004; 304: 714–718.

Tanzania Reproductive and Child Health Survey, 1999. Available at www.measuredhs.com.

UNAIDS. *UNAIDS/WHO AIDS Epidemic Update 2006.* Geneva: UNAIDS, 2006. Available at http://www.unaids.org/en/HIV_data/epi2006 (accessed 23 Jan 2007).

UNAIDS. *AIDS epidemic update 2005.* Geneva: UNAIDS, 2005a. Available at http://www.unaids.org/ Epi/2005/ (accessed 3 Jan 2006).

UNAIDS. *Evidence for HIV Decline in Zimbabwe: A Comprehensive Review of the Epidemiological Data.* Geneva: UNAIDS, 2005b. Available at http://data.unaids.org/ Publications/IRCpub06/Zimbabwe_Epi_report_Nov05_ en.pdf (accessed 2 Mar 2006).

UNFPA. *State of World Population 2005: The Promise of Equality: Gender Equity, Reproductive Health, and the Millennium Development Goals.* New York: UNFPA, 2005. Available at http://www.unfpa.org/swp/2005/pdf/ (accessed 18 May 2006).

United States Government Accountability Office. *GAO-06-395: Spending Requirement Presents Challenges for Allocating Prevention Funding under the President's Emergency Plan for AIDS Relief.* Washington, DC: GAO, April 2006.

United States Leadership Against HIV/AIDS, Tuberculosis, and Malaria Act of 2003 (HR 1298). Available at http://www. house.gov/pence/rsc/doc/rights%20under%20HIV-AIDS%20law.pdf (accessed 17 Mar 2006).

Wawer MJ, Gray R et al. *Declines in HIV Prevalence in Uganda: Not as Simple as ABC.* Presentation at Conference on Retroviruses and Opportunistic Infections, Boston, MA, 22 Feb 2005.

Weinhardt LS, Carey MP, Johnson BT, Bickham NL. Effects of HIV Counseling and Testing on Sexual Risk Behavior: A Meta-Analytic Review of Published Research, 1985–1997. *American Journal of Public Health* 1999; 89: 1397–1405.

Weller S, Davis K. Condom Effectiveness in Reducing Heterosexual HIV Transmission. *Cochrane Database Systematic Review* 2002; (1): CD003255.

Wilson D. *A Monitoring and Evaluation Framework for Concentrated Epidemics and Vulnerable Populations.* Washington, DC: The World Bank, 2005.

Wolitski R, MacGowan R, Higgins D, Jorgensen C. The Effects of HIV Counseling and Testing on Risk-Related Practices and Help-Seeking Behavior. *AIDS Education and Prevention* 1997; 9(Suppl B): 52–67.

Zambia Sexual Behavior Survey, 2003. Available at www.measuredhs.com.

Additional Relevant Studies

Genuis SJ, Genuis SK. Managing the Sexually Transmitted Disease Pandemic: A Time for Reevaluation. *American Journal of Obstetrics and Gynecology* 2004; 191: 1103–12.

Green, EC. Culture Clash and AIDS Prevention. *The Responsive Community* 2003; 13(4): 4–9.

Green EC, Witte K. Fear Arousal, Sexual Behavior Change and AIDS Prevention. *Journal of Health Communication,* 2006; 11:245-259. Available at http://www.gwu.edu/~cih/journal/JHClink/v11n3_green.pdf (accessed 8 Jan 2007).

Hendricks K (ed). *Evidence That Demands Action: Comparing Risk Avoidance and Risk Reduction strategies for HIV prevention.* Austin, TX: The Medical Institute for Sexual Health, 2004.

Low-Beer D. HIV-1 Incidence and Prevalence Trends in Uganda (Letter). *The Lancet* 2002; 360: 9347.

Low-Beer D, Stoneburner R. "Uganda and the Challenge of HIV/AIDS" in *The Political Economy of AIDS in Africa*, Poku N, Whiteside A (eds.). Aldershot, UK: Ashgate, 2004.

Moore DM, Hogg RS. Trends in Antenatal Human Immunodeficiency Virus Prevalence in Western Kenya and

Eastern Uganda: Evidence of Differences in Health Policies? *International Journal of Epidemiology* 2004; 33: 542–548.

Muhwezi J. Uganda HIV/AIDS Sero-Behavioural Survey 2004–05 Preliminary Report. Kampala, Uganda: Ministry of Health, June 2005.

Richens J, Imrie J, Weiss H. Sex and Death: Why Does HIV Continue to Spread When So Many People Know About the Risks? *Journal of the Royal Statistical Society Series A*; 2003; 166: 207–215.

Shelton JD. Partner Reduction Remains the Predominant Explanation (Letter). *British Medical Journal* 2005; 330: 496.